Yackety Yack
- Let's Talk Backs.
...and more!

Alicia Leontieff & Wendy Davis

CONTENTS

INTRODUCTION:
1
ABOUT THE AUTHORS

CHAPTER ONE:
7
WHAT ARE THE DIFFERENT DISCIPLINES?

CHAPTER TWO:
15
A CHIROPRACTIC COURSE OF CARE

CHAPTER THREE:
27
STOP STRESSING

CHAPTER FOUR.
50
POSTURE PERFECT

CHAPTER FIVE:
63
X-RAYS

CHAPTER SIX:
75
HERE COMES THE SCIENCE BIT / THE HEALING PROCESS TAKES TIME

CHAPTER SEVEN:
88
YOU ARE WHAT YOU EAT

CHAPTER EIGHT:
101
EXERCISE CAN BE BAD FOR YOU

CHAPTER NINE:
112
SURGERY SHOULD BE THE LAST RESORT

INTRODUCTION:
ABOUT THE AUTHORS

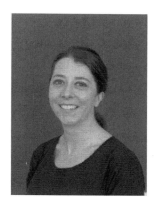

Alicia Leontieff was born in Manchester. At the age of 12, she injured her back falling off a tree swing from a considerable height. It was then that her mother, Pat, a great believer in complimentary therapies, decided to take her to an Osteopath to address the problem. After an intensive course of care, she had eliminated not only her lower back problems, but also her dependence upon wrist supports (she'd suffered a skiing fracture several years earlier). She also discovered that her recurrent throat infections, with which she had suffered for many years, had vanished. Both Pat and Alicia were so grateful for the care she had received, that it was natural for Alicia to choose a career that involved helping people. Having looked into the many different branches of the healthcare field, Alicia felt drawn to Chiropractic.

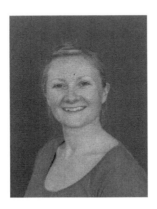

Wendy Davis was born in South Africa to British parents. At the age of 12, she and her mother returned to the UK after the unexpected death of her father. As a child, Wendy witnessed Chiropractic care first hand, observing her mum's treatment for recurring neck problems. This experience planted the seeds that would result in her decision to become a Chiropractor and attend Glamorgan University (now called The University of South Wales) for the intensive four-year degree course. It was there that Alicia and Wendy met. They realised early on that they had similar thoughts, shared core values, and had the same vision: running a practice full of happy and healthy people.

In 2006, they acquired a small practice in Bury, Lancashire, which was originally called Meridian Chiropractic. Over the years that followed, the practice grew and grew, culminating in their move from a small building accessed through four flights of stairs, to a 1,600 square-foot building set over three floors. The practice now has an on-site digital x-ray suite, computerised orthotics equipment and a great team of Chiropractors, massage therapists and Chiropractic assistants, all there to serve the community, helping them to regain and maintain their passion for life by fulfilling their true vitality, health potential and wellbeing.

Alicia and Wendy share a love of the ocean and the beach, and have incorporated its calming colour scheme into the centre's aesthetics. With their high standards, their practice exudes quality, including its surroundings, customer service, and products. Alicia, Wendy and their specially selected team ensure that the service all their guests receive is consistently exceptional. Team work and team development are key when delivering a world-class service, and to that end, they hold regular team coaching sessions and self-development sessions.

So, what inspired us to write this book?

In the United Kingdom we currently have the NHS, (National Health Service), which makes healthcare easily accessible. It has served our country well over the years, providing essential services to all, regardless of circumstance. As further advances to healthcare are made, we are living longer. Great! But there is a catch - with people living longer, the NHS has to support more and more people, and we see an ever-ageing population.

With funding tending to come from central government, resources are becoming increasingly stretched, placing great strain on medical professionals and patients alike. We felt we were hearing too many stories of people being denied expensive but potentially life-saving treatments because of the expense. Why was this allowed to happen when others were receiving what we believed to be unnecessary treatments at substantial costs? It all seemed such an unfair waste of resources and became a source of frustration for us.

We have seen thousands of people over the years taking cocktails of drugs for chronic conditions, for symptoms such as lower back pain, gastric reflux, headaches, migraines, sciatica, hip pain, and irritable bowel syndrome (IBS). They would have been on these drugs for years, we believed unnecessarily, as a result of not being given either the opportunity or the correct information to help themselves.

Medication is costing the NHS millions of pounds every year, and, in most cases, causes unnecessary side effects for the people taking them. Further medication is often required to counter those problems. This may then result in additional side effects from these additional drugs, more medication for *those*, and the cycle continues until people find themselves on a cocktail of drugs.

We have also seen many people that we believed to have been recommended unnecessary operations, such as hip and knee replacements and spinal operations, because they had simply neglected aches and pains for years without seeking any help. Eventually their pain became intolerable and the area so degenerative that an operation was inevitable. Had they sought help or been offered it when the problem had originally started, we believe surgery may have been avoidable. These operations cost the taxpayer a considerable amount of money, running into thousands of pounds per patient. We believe that most surgeries could have been avoided with a more proactive approach to health.

Don't get us wrong —the care that the NHS provides is wonderful. For life-threatening conditions and emergencies, our health service is second-to-none. If you need emergency surgery, the medics are there straight away, concerned only about your health and wellbeing rather than wanting your insurance details and assessing your ability to pay. With fractured bones and accidents, the NHS really does come into its own. Accident and Emergency is the NHS's niche and is what it excels at. What we believe it isn't so wonderful with, is dealing with chronic conditions. It doesn't have the resources —the personnel, the time or money— to thoroughly correct all patients' conditions. There has to be a time and session limit for each person seen by the NHS; remember that there are thousands of others also waiting to be seen for their problems, too. If treatment is not thorough enough, the original problem never completely resolves and can often progress to further areas.

For example, if you sprained your ankle and couldn't walk, you may make an appointment to see your GP. By the time you receive treatment your acute (new) problem has become a chronic problem (something that has been there for months). You may be recommended physiotherapy, and after a few sessions, the pain may subside. However, what may not have been addressed is the impact your sprained ankle — restricting your normal walking pattern over weeks— has had on the rest of your body. This may now have caused a knee problem. However, this knee problem isn't impacting your life too much yet, and has therefore gone unmentioned to your practitioner, who may not have had time to look at the rest of your body, or your knee, when assessing the ankle. This can become a ticking time bomb, leading to knee or hip degeneration, and even lower back pain. Had you been assessed thoroughly enough at the start then this potential knee problem, or the resulting degeneration, could have been averted. The same for the resulting hip and lower back pain. It's these knock-on effects which now need addressing, which we believe places further but avoidable strain on our wonderful NHS. We feel it's happening all too often.

Let's consider this: are headaches or lower back pain the result of an aspirin shortage? No! Had those in pain considered WHY their symptoms existed in the first place and addressed the matter thoroughly when those symptoms first arose, then taking drugs and suffering was a path they may need not have travelled.

We believe that because healthcare is free in the UK, many people don't place a high enough value on it; we are very fortunate to be able to take a "free" trip to the GP followed by a visit to the pharmacist, for often heavily-subsidised medication.

Take lower back pain for instance, this alone costs the NHS millions of pounds in care every year and is detrimental to our economy due to time spent off work, resulting in decreased productivity nationwide. We believe this could be avoided by promoting a more forward-thinking approach to health and wellbeing, doing a few daily stretches, and being proactive rather than reactive. The alternative, taking some tablets and then waiting for the pain to subside, does not address the cause. A proactive approach could also serve to avoid or alleviate stress and depression, as well as a whole host of other symptoms.

We believe there are ways to combat this, things that you can do which will not only empower you to be more productive and feel better, but also to live happier fulfilling lives with fewer trips to the Doctor's Surgery.

We would like to help you understand how to become more proactive about your health. We hope to give you alternatives so that you can become less reliant on unnecessary medications that only mask the symptoms rather than truly correcting them, and start thinking about why a problem or symptom is there and what you can do to be rid of it. There is so much you can do to help yourself. In the words of Dr James Chestnut (international speaker, author and Chiropractor), by thinking well, moving well and eating well, you can affect your health and well-being for the better!

CHAPTER 1:
WHAT ARE THE DIFFERENT DISCIPLINES?

We are often asked what the differences are between Chiropractic, Osteopathy, Acupuncture, and Physiotherapy.

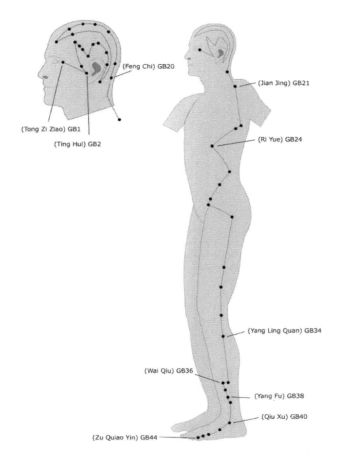

Diagram showing an example of one of the meridian lines

used in acupuncture.

Acupuncture is based on the premise that the body contains meridian lines, or lines where energy, or Qi, flows. These lines don't tend to be connected anatomically. If a meridian line becomes blocked anywhere along its pathway this can affect the flow of energy, or Qi, resulting in dysfunction and symptoms such as pain, for example.

The Acupuncturist's job is to work out where these energy lines are being blocked, gently tap a thin, disposable needle into the area to re-establish energy flow, and thus restore Qi. Like Chiropractic, Acupuncture can be used to prevent symptoms from recurring.

Dry needling is often confused with Acupuncture, although the two are not interchangeable. Practitioners such as Osteopaths, Physiotherapists and Chiropractors tend to use dry needling to compliment the work they already do. Disposable needles are used in dry needling- the same as the ones used in Acupuncture- but these needles generally aren't inserted into blocked energy lines - like they are in Acupuncture - but rather, into trigger points in muscles to reduce pain. Practitioners can generally learn how to dry needle in a weekend, whereas Acupuncturists are qualified to degree level in the UK, and train for years to perfect their art.

What are trigger points?

Trigger points are localised areas of muscle tightness. When the nerve supply to a muscle is compromised, muscles can become tight, and areas of scar tissue can form within them. These areas are often referred to as muscle "knots," and these knots can cause pain. Trigger points are muscle "knots" that can refer pain towards other parts of the body. For example, there are muscles located around the shoulder that can become tight and often contain trigger points which can then refer symptoms such as pain, numbness and tingling into the arms. One theory for the mechanism behind trigger point referral patterns is that those patterns are linked to areas that were once connected during the embryonic stages. So using the example of the shoulder —during your body's early development— cells of the shoulder and arm were located immediately next to each other, *in utero*, and as your body grows, they still maintain their embryonic connections, thus enabling them to refer to each other.

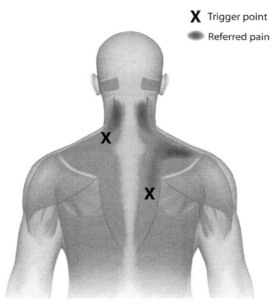

Diagram showing an example of a trigger point and how it refers pain away from the site.

Pressing on trigger points, or inserting a dry needle into them, results in increased blood flow to the area, enabling the body to heal itself and break down these areas of scar tissue. This is also the premise by which soft tissue massage works.

This is not to be confused with Acupressure! Acupressure is a technique similar in principle to Acupuncture, and involves placing pressure onto blocked energy, or Qi lines. The aim is to clear blockages in the body and restore Qi. Pressure may be applied by the hand, or by the elbow. Interestingly, some of the traditional Acupressure spots can be found to overlap common trigger point sites.

Physiotherapists tend to focus and work within a localised area of the body. For example, if they are treating a shoulder problem, they tend to work only on the shoulder, and they may incorporate some work on the neck into their treatments. Physios wouldn't normally tend to work on the body as a whole. They do provide exercises for their patients as well as giving advice on things they can do at home to better manage their symptoms. Physiotherapists may also use massage to break down scar tissue and trigger points. Some Physiotherapists will use modalities, for example an ultrasound machine, to help speed up the healing process. Ultrasound has been used by Physiotherapists since the 1940s and has been shown to accelerate healing times by increasing blood flow to the damaged area and reducing pain.

Some Physiotherapists specialise in manipulation. They grade the manipulations that they do, and the types they use. Their manipulations tend to involve joint "springing" (repetitive pushing on the same joint) to mobilise and loosen up the jammed area. Manipulations tend to be taught in post-graduate courses and take place over a series of weekends. Many Physiotherapists work within the National Health Service. NHS Physiotherapists usually acquire their patients via a consultant or GP and follow their diagnosis. Physiotherapists then work on the area specified by the GP or consultant using a set number of visits and protocols, discharging patients as soon as possible. Some Physiotherapists work privately, so they have more autonomy, and tend to design bespoke care plans to treat an area.

Osteopathy originated in the USA and was founded by Andrew Taylor Still in 1895. The philosophy behind Osteopathy is, historically speaking, based on increasing blood flow to an area to aid healing. If an area of the body becomes jammed, it can disturb the flow of blood and thus result in unfavourable symptoms. Osteopaths use a range of adjustments, mobilisations and soft tissue therapies or massage, to work on blocked or jammed areas to restore function.

An Osteopath's initial training does not tend to cover radiography, and therefore they are not trained to take X-rays, even though they are educated to degree level. As a patient, we believe that you wouldn't notice much difference between what an Osteopath does and what a Chiropractor does. Both use slightly different techniques and are based on different principles. Chiropractors tend to utilise X-rays more frequently, which we believe helps us create a more bespoke care plan and hence provide a more accurate diagnosis and prognosis for the patient.

Chiropractic comes from the Greek word "Kheir," meaning *hand,* and "practic," meaning practice. Chiropractic, like Osteopathy, originated in the USA, and was founded in 1896. Its founding Father was Daniel David Palmer. The history books tell us of how he adjusted the mid back of a deaf janitor, Harvey Lillard, and by doing so, cured his deafness.

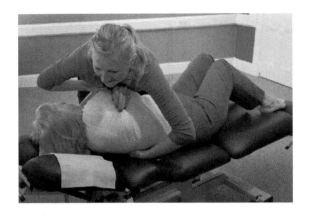

Image of Wendy adjusting a similar area.

Palmer's son, BJ, continued to develop the profession. As the profession grew and Chiropractic care became increasingly popular, Chiropractors were prosecuted and jailed for practising medicine without a licence. However, the premise of Chiropractic care is that the body heals itself and that Chiropractors don't actually "treat" anything. Rather, they work on restoring normal movement to jammed areas which are causing nerve interference in the body, producing symptoms such as pain. Restoring normal movement to an area corrects nerve flow which allows the body to heal itself. It was this premise which eventually freed those jailed Chiropractors as they could truthfully state they were not practising medicine; rather, they were enabling the body to do what it does best: heal itself.

Chiropractors tend to choose to adjust more than Osteopaths. An adjustment is a way of loosening up a stuck joint (gently by hand) to enable the body to heal itself and restore normal function. During an adjustment, clicks and pops may be heard. This is the movement of air into and out of the joint.

Chiropractors use adjustments as opposed to manipulations.

An adjustment has a more focused intent, whereas a manipulation has a more general application. We choose to use the word *adjustment* over *manipulation,* as it is our philosophy to maintain positivity at all times. The word "manipulation," to us, has a negative feel; for example, people "manipulate" numbers and figures. Manipulations can be taught over the course of a weekend, whereas adjustments involve years and years of practice and refinement. To be able to move a stuck joint from A to B with finesse is not only a skill but an art form forged over time.

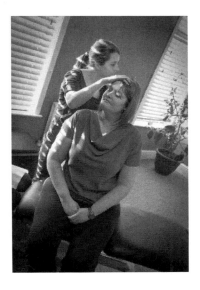

In the image above, Alicia uses her hands to find restrictions in the neck.

With adjustments, clicks or pops may be heard. This is the sound of the release of gas bubbles within the joint. However, Chiropractic adjustments have been proven to be over one thousand times safer than taking an aspirin. Back in the day, old wives tales publicised the theory that the clicking and popping of joints caused arthritis. However, the opposite is true. Adjusting a jammed area and restoring correct nerve function to that area has been shown to slow down degeneration.

A study by DeWeber, Olszewski & Ortolano (2011) looked at degeneration in the hands of people who cracked their knuckles compared to the degeneration in those that didn't. They found that the "knuckle-crackers" had no more degeneration than those who did not crack their knuckles and, in fact, cite studies which found the reverse to be true; those who knuckle-cracked had *less* degeneration than those who didn't.

Osteomyologists will often have studied as Chiropractors or Osteopaths before becoming frustrated with their respective governing bodies. Eventually, they formed a combined and inclusive new profession, whose practitioners can practice more autonomously. The term Osteomyology was derived from the words "Osteo" meaning *bone*, "myo" meaning *muscle*, and "ology," meaning *study*, and was coined in 1992 by Dr Sir Alan Clemens, who was originally an Osteopath.

Chapter summary:

Acupuncture and dry needling are not the same. Chiropractors, Osteopaths and Physiotherapists are all educated to degree standards. Physiotherapists tend to be more localised in their approach and commonly use modalities to help them. Chiropractors and Osteopaths approach health holistically. Chiropractors take and analyse X- Rays which can provide the patient with a more accurate diagnosis, prognosis and care plan. The premise of Chiropractic care is that the body heals itself.

CHAPTER 2:
A CHIROPRACTIC COURSE OF CARE

People often ask whether Chiropractic care could help them because they have x, y, z, or worry that they are too old, or too young. There is also an assumption that we can't help because they've had an operation on the area, or because they've been told nothing can be done for them. Our reply is that you are ALWAYS better off with a spine and nervous system that functions well rather than one that doesn't, regardless of age, operations, or pre-existing conditions.

Nothing happens in your body without a signal from the brain running through the spinal cord and out through the nerves. The nerves in your body are linked to everything; every tissue, muscle and organ.

The spine and skull house the central nervous system. If the spine and/or any single vertebrae becomes stuck, swelling can cause the nerves to become pinched. Irritation of the nerve often results in a symptom somewhere along the path that particular nerve supplies. So you could say that a bone out of place pinches a nerve and causes a problem. If that particular bone or vertebrae is adjusted back into its correct place, and retrained to stay put, the pressure is taken off the nerve, allowing the body to heal itself, thereby rectifying the problem. We believe Chiropractic care therefore gives life to your years and adds years to your life.

The diagram below shows the spine, where the nerves come from and what areas of the body those nerves supply.

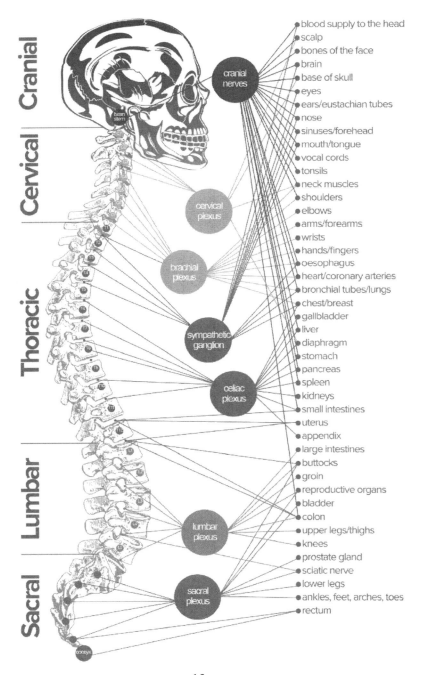

Whilst mainstream medicine tends to focus on the area of pain and treat that one area, Chiropractors look at the body as a whole and how the entire body is moving and functioning. The body should move like a well-oiled machine; degeneration in one area might not necessarily be coming from the area that is jammed. A useful analogy for this is the wheel alignment of a car. If the wheels aren't aligned, you will get excess wear on the tyres. If the body isn't aligned, wear and tear can manifest in one particular spot, e.g. the hip or knee. Just addressing the knee or hip will not prevent further degeneration in those areas as the original problem wasn't with the knee or the hip, but with the misaligned spine. Re-aligning the entire body helps to prevent excessive pressure on both the knees and hips, thereby relieving pain and slowing the degenerative process. Chiropractic care is holistic, it works on the body as a whole.

When someone comes to see us for the first time or when they make that first phone call, we find they have four key questions on their minds.

Firstly, *"what is wrong with me?"* The consultation and examination is designed to work out exactly what is causing the symptoms by utilising neurological and orthopaedic tests, in combination with x-rays if deemed necessary. This helps us to work out how much degeneration is present in an area and whether a vertebrae or joint is misaligned or jammed.

Secondly, *"how can you help me?"* We like to spend a lot of time explaining how we can help you. We use a variety of techniques that have been shown to be a thousand times safer than taking an aspirin, and so safe that you are more likely to be hit by lightning twice than suffer severe consequences from a Chiropractic adjustment. It is one of the safest forms of care around, and is statistically safer than any form of medication you may take or operation you could have. It is statistically safer than travelling in a plane or in your car.

With Chiropractic care enabling the body to heal itself, symptoms that have been present for many months, or even years, can begin to subside, the amount of medications taken can be reduced, sleep patterns can improve, and energy levels can be restored as well as mobility.

A study by an American Insurance company found that families who utilise Chiropractic care use far fewer medical services. They found that hospital admissions were down by 60%, hospital stays were down by 69%, outpatient procedures were down by 85% and that pharmaceutical use was down by 56%.

Thirdly, *"how long is it going to take to get me out of pain and to get me right?"* This is always dependant on the individual. There are so many factors that can influence the healing process. For example: How long the problem has been there, and the amount of degeneration present are both factors that will affect the speed at which you heal. For those who smoke, the healing process will take longer.

Those who drink plenty of water as opposed to caffeine-laden drinks such as coffee and tea will heal more quickly. The same is true for those who eat plenty of fruit and vegetables and have a varied diet, as they are providing their body with all the nutrients it needs to heal, as opposed to those who have a takeaway every night and favour carbohydrates. The correct lifestyle and ergonomics also play important roles in the recovery process. Office workers who sit all day and barely move around, sitting hunched over a screen, will take longer to heal than those who are more active.

How effective the adjustment is and how long it holds, is determined by the length of time in between adjustments and what you are actually doing in between your appointments. For example, people who keep to the frequency of their recommended care plan, keep to their appointments and do the things they are asked to do, respond best to care. This may include stretches and core exercises, along with making the suggested changes to their lifestyle. It's also important to heed advice on what not to do; such as being advised not to start back at the gym too early, or not to go training for a marathon too soon.

According to the American Academy of Orthopaedic Surgeons, damaging a joint raises the chances of developing arthritis in that area sevenfold. So incidences such as road traffic accidents, slips and falls which can cause areas to become jammed or locked, should always be treated seriously and addressed quickly. The sooner an area is adjusted, the less chance it has of arthritic changes developing.

Lastly, *"how much will it cost?"* How much a course of care will cost is again dependant upon how long the problem has been there, and what it actually is. We have known people who could not initially afford care return to us at a later date having saved up. It's better to wait a few extra months to sort something that has been there a long time, than never start at all. We take more care looking after our mobile phones and tablets, putting them down to recharge every night, than we do our bodies. When do we allow our own bodies to recharge? We brush our teeth twice a day to prevent decay. We service our car and MOT it. Phones and tablets can be replaced, teeth can be filled or replaced. What are you doing to help your spine and nervous system, to prevent decay in your joints? Our spine and nervous system cannot be replaced. We have to look after them, and make the most of the bodies we have.

Your body is the most amazing piece of equipment you will ever own. Health is the most valuable asset we possess and we must treasure it above all else.

Everyone who attends a health centre should be told before committing to care - as they are with us-what we have found, whether we can help, how long it will take, and how much it will cost.

Why do Chiropractors focus on the spine and nervous system?

We believe the role of the nervous system on the body is often overlooked by both health care professionals and the public in general. It's vital that the nervous system is functioning at its best. Everything in your body has a nerve supply: every tissue, muscle, and organ. Nothing happens in the body without a signal from the brain running through the spinal cord and out through the nerves. It has been shown that the weight of a 5p coin on a nerve can disrupt the flow of nervous information by up to 60 per cent, and you wouldn't necessarily know about it, or even feel it.

The nerves from the lower back go down the legs and towards the abdomen. They supply the bladder and bowels, the buttocks, the hips, the groin, the thighs and legs, the knees, the shins, the calves and the feet. If any of the nerves are irritated in the lower back by a vertebrae that's stuck and swollen or a disc that's bulged, symptoms can occur in any one of those parts of the body.

For example, IBS-type symptoms such as constipation, diarrhoea and bloating can occur when the nerves in the lower back are being pinched. Period pains can also be the result of nerves being irritated in the lower back, as the nerves from the lower back go to the uterus. Hip pain can be the result of lower back dysfunction, as the nerves which serve the hip also come from the lower back.

Shortly after taking over a previous Chiropractor's patient, we were having a conversation with a lady explaining how the nerves which come from the lower back supply the bladder and bowels, and how irritation of the nerves can often result in dysfunction in those areas. She started to tell me about one of her sons, who was aged ten at the time, and who was wetting the bed nightly. He was very anxious about it and wanted to go away on overnight school trips but felt too embarrassed to. She wondered whether we could help, as she had exhausted all other options. We examined her son's spine to see how well his nervous system was functioning, and located spots where the spine was jammed, irritating the nerves. We believed that this was affecting the flow of information from the bladder to the brain and from the brain to the bladder. Thereby the signal was being lost or delayed when the bladder wanted to let the brain know that it was full and needed emptying. After a good course of care which concentrated on removing the nerve interference, the son responded really nicely and after a few months, his bed was never wet again.

Sciatica is something we have seen thousands of times and have had great success with. This is caused when the sciatic nerve in the lower back becomes irritated or "pinched," resulting in leg pain. Knee pain is not always caused solely by problems with the knee joint itself but can also come from your lower back. The Femoral and Obturator nerves supply the knee and come from the lower back. It therefore stands to reason that your knee pain could be the result of pressure on these nerves in the lower part of the back and not with the knee joint at all. Other symptoms which can also occur as a result of nerves being irritated in the lower back include, but are not limited to, shin pains, calf pains and plantar fasciitis.

If the nerve supply to an area is compromised, the area that nerve supplies will become stuck and can then degenerate. The actual cause of the degeneration is not the stuck or jammed joint but rather the compromised nerve supply *to* that area or joint.

If we treat a person who complains of hip pain without looking at the nerve supply (which comes from the lower back) to the hip, we will never yield perfect results. Chiropractors will work on removing the nerve irritation to the symptomatic area by adjusting the spine, allowing the body to heal itself, repair the damage and resolve the symptoms.

The nerves from the mid back (or thoracic spine) serve the vital organs, the heart and lungs, the rib cage, and the digestive organs such as the liver, stomach, and pancreas. If nerves are being irritated in the mid back by a vertebrae that is stuck or mis-aligned, those areas could be affected by this reduction in nervous information. We have seen symptoms such as indigestion, heartburn, reflux, asthma, and the inability to inhale deeply, be the result of a jammed mid-back. People often have tests to work out the exact cause of these symptoms but more often than not, the impact of the thoracic spine on these organs is overlooked, particularly in cases where the test results have come back as "normal."

In other cases, where things such as hiatus hernias are found, we wonder what caused the hernia to be there; what has caused that weakness? We believe that an irritated nerve to this area will have had a massive impact on how the organs function, resulting in weakness, dysfunction and inevitable symptoms. The patient is often prescribed medication for the resulting digestive symptoms, such as antacids like omeprazole, which can cause problems and result in other medications being prescribed for the resultant side effects. This can become a slippery slope, and once you are on it, it can inevitably end up with you having to take a small bag of medications each and every day for life. Chiropractors will work on removing the nerve irritation in the mid back by adjusting the jammed area, allowing the body to heal itself, removing the likely cause of the symptoms rather than just the symptom itself.

The nerves from the neck go to the head and face, to the shoulder, to the chest, diaphragm and down the arms to the elbows, wrists and fingertips. If the nerves are irritated in the neck by a vertebrae that is stuck, it can affect the flow of nervous information to any and all of the above areas, resulting in dysfunction and/or pain. By removing the nerve interference in the neck, by adjusting the jammed vertebrae and freeing it up, increasing the nerve supply to these areas, we enable the body to heal itself.

Often, people think that adjusting a joint just once or twice, which has been stuck for a long time, resulting in degeneration and nerve irritation, will resolve an issue that has been present for months, years, or in a lot of cases, decades. Sadly, this is not so. The healing process takes time. An area that has been stuck for a while will not move freely after just a handful of adjustments.

Each time a jammed joint is adjusted, the tendency is for the joint to go back to its old habits and get stuck again. The body likes habit and it does *not* like change. Additionally, the lifestyle that brought about the dysfunction in the first place does not just go away between adjustments, which results in the tightening up again of the stuck area. It is therefore imperative that a sufficient and robust course of care is recommended. The period of time between each adjustment is critical; this, combined with what the patient's lifestyle is like between adjustments, has a massive effect on how long the vertebrae stays mobile before tightening back up again.

In the initial stages of a care plan, the adjustments need to be close together and frequent to encourage the body and stuck areas to become loose and stay loose. The surrounding areas then need to be strengthened in order for the adjustments to continue to hold in the future, then more and more activities can be reintroduced into daily life. We liken a course of care to that of training for a marathon. You wouldn't start off straight away running 26 miles, you would start off by walking around the block and gradually increasing your journey each time, until you are running your desired distance. The same can be said for a course of care. You start to introduce adjustments to the spine, changes in lifestyle, stretches and core exercises, massage and orthotics (bespoke foot arch supports for your shoes) over a period of time, introducing things slowly, easing the body into this new and improved state, encouraging it to stay loose whilst removing the nerve irritation. Soft tissue damage (such as ligaments and nerves) can take up to two years to heal —and in our experience a **<u>minimum</u>** of three months. This process cannot be bypassed, and doesn't differ massively from person-to-person, so it is imperative that a course of care lasts a minimum of three months to allow enough time for healing to take place and to make sure that once everything is fully repaired, the body is in tip-top shape.

We have seen thousands of people over the years with a variety of symptoms and problems. The vast majority have responded extremely well to care, and there are many cases which stand out. We have helped people who have been in so much pain that they have told us we were their last resort, and they had been considering ending it all as they were so depressed.

The manner in which the body functions and heals is amazing. The body is made to heal itself, and it should not require medications or surgery to do this. All it needs is a positive mindset, the correct diet, and an optimal functioning nervous system and brain, and it will do what it needs to do. Chiropractic adjustments are vital to free up any nervous system irritation. Be proactive and seek help. It is never too late. The earlier you seek help, the better. You only get one spine and one nervous system and they cannot be replaced, so make the most of the body you have! We have seen massive degenerative changes in spines where symptoms have been neglected for just two years. Imagine what a difference could have been made to those people's lives had they sought help straight away. Conversely, imagine what could have happened if they had neglected their symptoms for a further five, ten, or even fifteen years! The number of degenerative changes that we believe would have taken place over such a period of time would be massive, and the impact those changes would have had on the body could be catastrophic. Don't allow this to happen to you. Take responsibility for our own health. Exercise, eat well, think well, and enjoy Chiropractic care. It's never too late, nor too early to begin.

Chapter summary:

The nervous system controls everything in the body. The spine houses the nervous system. If the spine is not functioning correctly it can impact on everything and anything. Chiropractors are holistic and look at locating areas of spinal and joint dysfunction and adjust them restoring correct nerve flow, allowing the body to heal itself. When people attend our centre, they will know what is causing their problem, how we can help, how long it will take and how much it will cost before committing to care.

The nerves from the neck supply the head, shoulders and arms, the nerves from the mid-back supply the vital and digestive organs, and the nerves from the lower back supply the bladder and bowels, legs, hips, knees and feet. If there is any irritation to any nerve, dysfunction or disease ensues. Make the most of your spine and nervous system. It cannot be replaced. It is never too late or too early to begin care.

CHAPTER 3:
STOP STRESSING

In our line of work as Chiropractors, we enjoy spending time not only helping our patients get well but also being engaged with what's going on in their lives. For some, lending an impartial ear and offering an alternative view point is invaluable. In this role of unofficial "psychiatrist," we hear over and over again that we are all leading busy —and sometimes stressful— lives.

But what is "stress"? Well, firstly, we would say that there are three distinct and different categories. The first one we are going to touch on is "Emotional stress". This is what we would say most people are referring to when they say they are feeling "stressed out." But there are an additional two categories that you may not have considered, or even heard of, and these are "chemical" and "physical" stress or stresses.

EMOTIONAL STRESS

Most people will recognise the causes of emotional stress and can relate to them. For example, your alarm clock fails to wake you, you get up late, you nearly trip down the stairs half-dressed with your hair still wet from the shower. In your haste to bolt down your morning brew, you scold your tongue. Cursing, you leave the house only to return five seconds later to check you've locked the front door. You jump in your car and manage to trap your coat in the car door, reopen the door, rescue your coat, get back inside the car, and drive off. You grit your teeth as you hit all the red traffic lights between home and work and arrive just in time for your boss to check on you. You're late! Most people would agree that this was a "stressful" start to your day!

So what is occurring in your body whilst all this happening? As your brain gets stressed, it sends a signal to your adrenal glands to produce more adrenaline. This is your "fight or flight" response, and is your body's way of getting you away from danger as fast as possible. Your heart rate and blood pressure rise, and you may start to sweat; your pupils will also dilate. The body secretes the stress hormone, cortisol, from the adrenal cortex of the adrenal gland. Cortisol is a hormone which, amongst other things, increases the rate at which sugar/energy is released into your bloodstream. Long-term or chronic exposure to high levels of adrenaline and cortisol have been linked to increased anxiety, depression, digestion problems, headaches, heart disease, sleep problems, weight gain and difficulties with memory recall and concentration.

Your mood, or feelings, can also affect your posture. Think of someone you know who is joyful, confident and full of life. I bet that when they stand next to you, one of the first things you'll notice is that they have their shoulders back, chest out and head upright (think of an exclamation mark!) Conversely, think of someone you care about, or even yourself, someone who is stressed, "under the weather," and miserable. Your posture, or theirs, may resemble that of a question mark; that of someone with rounded shoulders, slumped posture with their head in a more forward position.

A gentleman walked into our centre one day. He was miserable and had been having terrible, electric-like shooting pains down his right leg for over a month, ever since he had slipped off his roof trying to put up his Christmas lights. His wife couldn't believe it when she saw him tumble past the kitchen window as she was doing the washing up! He came in with terrible pain but was also depressed, because he was a professional, self-employed, driveway installer. This meant that on the run-up to Christmas, not only was he in pain, but he wasn't working. Not working meant that he was not getting paid. Not getting paid meant that Christmas for his young family was going to be tight.

Now, because this gentleman was feeling pretty low, he had adopted this "unhappy posture." This meant his shoulders were hunched and his head was slumped forward, so, in addition to the back and leg pain, he was beginning to experience burning neck pains as well! This was no surprise when you consider that the average head weighs ten pounds, and for every inch your chin moves forward, the weight of your head increases by a pound due to the downward force of gravity. If you don't believe us, try this little experiment when you are next at the ten-pin bowling alley. Pick up a ten-pound ball and hold it out in front of you at arms' length. This represents the weight of your head when it's forward. See how long it takes for your arms to feel the strain. This is what is happening to your neck and shoulder muscles when your head is in this forward position. Compare this to how long you are able to hold the bowling ball comfortably when it's close to your chest. This represents the weight of your head in its correct position, balancing nicely on top of your neck bones and not placing so much strain on the neck and shoulder muscles. We will be talking more about posture in the next chapter.

If you were wondering how the gentleman got on, he responded fabulously to care and his family had a great Christmas!

Poor sleep

We see lots of people who suffer from emotional stress, and one of the most common symptoms they experience is poor sleep. We are told that it can be difficult to drift off to sleep, because you are allowing your brain to chatter away to you, reminding you of all the things you didn't get done today and all the things you need to remember to do tomorrow. Or, you can wake early in the morning, mulling over what you didn't get done yesterday, and worrying about all those jobs, meetings and responsibilities that you now need to catch up with today. You are scared that you will forget, that you won't remember what it was that your brain was twittering on about before you went to sleep the night before. This can be so frustrating for many. Unfortunately if you allow this to happen regularly, it trains your brain to accept this behaviour as necessary and normal and this will, in future, prevent you from either nodding off, or, conversely, wake you in the small hours of the morning. Studies tell us that sleep is extremely important for our health and cell repair and that the average adult should be aiming for about eight hours of uninterrupted sleep a night. Something that we have found to be very useful in combatting "brain chatter" is to use a notepad, or some people may prefer to keep a diary. The key thing, however, is to write down all your thoughts, stressful things and those "must dos" and "don't forgets" for the coming days and weeks. If you do this an hour before you go to bed, it can reduce the time you spend trying to fall asleep by up to 50 percent. You are now giving your brain permission to switch off. Do this every night for a month and watch your sleep patterns improve.

Bedtime routine

Another tried and tested method for training your body to prepare for sleep is something that our mothers (and most likely yours, too) trained you to do from a very early age and that is to have a set bedtime routine, from which you rarely deviate. So, for example, when Wendy was a little child, this was her routine: Dinner was about 6pm, and at about 7pm, her Mum would start telling her to have a bath. Wendy is a night owl and always has been, so she would stretch this out to about 7:30pm. After bath time, it was pyjamas on, brush teeth, go to the toilet and be tucked up in bed by 8pm. Regardless of it being a school day or a weekend, this was the routine. Her body knew it well, and by 8:05, Wendy would be sound asleep.

We realise that having the exact same bedtime routine and morning routine every day is not always possible, but if you can stick to it as best you can then you will eventually program your body to drift off to sleep. Make sure that you stay well hydrated by drinking filtered tap water throughout the day. Try and breathe through your nose more; you will conserve water. This ensures that you won't wake up in the middle of the night with a dry mouth, gasping for water. If you exercise more during the day, then you should also sleep better at night. We will go on to talk more about exercise in chapter 8.

Another symptom of emotional stress that you may not even be aware of is "jaw clenching." The muscles that control the jaw are called the muscles of mastication (you work these muscles when you chew your food) and when you clench your jaw, you also activate these muscle groups. Some studies have shown that chewing or clenching on one side can affect the function of the jaw, which can then adversely affect the neck. So if you are having to eat on one side because of a problem with one of your teeth, try not to put off the necessary dental work needed.

Studies have also found a significant correlation between poor neck posture and jaw dysfunction, particularly when tenderness was reported in the trapezius muscle (a muscle found in the neck) and the temporalis muscle (one of the chewing muscles). This tenderness can result in poor posture and cause the upper neck bones to become misaligned. The change in posture can cause the lower jaw to protrude forward and can lead to an improper bite. Having an improper bite is one of the leading causes of temporomandibular joint (jaw) pain. So, having correct posture can be the key to solving jaw problems. We will explore correct posture in chapter 4.

This reminds us about a conversation we had with one of our patients, who was in her fifties and came to see us with chronic neck pain and headaches. She was one of life's high flyers and would spend two to four hours every day, Monday to Friday, driving her beloved Mini up and down the M6 motorway in her role as trouble-shooter for a large supermarket chain. It was a role she loved, but she was becoming more and more frustrated with the stresses involved in driving, from traffic jams to road rage and everything in between. She didn't realise (but we did), that as soon as she drove onto that motorway, she would brace herself and grit her teeth for all those inevitable challenges. She would grit those teeth and tense that jaw all the way up and down that motorway. Over the years, this had caused an imbalance in her jaw muscles and it was this that was contributing to her neck pain and headaches.

Being made aware that you clench your teeth is key in helping to correct it. If you do clench, try to adopt a more relaxed jaw position with your mouth slightly open when you drive. Once she learned to do this, and combined with a course of Chiropractic care, which included both neck and jaw adjustments, she felt so much more at ease and better able to cope with her daily commute.

CHEMICAL STRESS

Another type of stress is chemical stress. By this, we mean the chemicals we physically come into contact with or ingest on a regular basis. Your body is amazing at processing and getting rid of the large majority of these. But continuous, regular and/or excessive quantities can be too much for the body and lead to "toxic overload."

There are so many things we should be either avoiding

completely or at least minimising contact with, that this alone is a subject for another book. So we have just decided to concentrate on the most common chemical stresses, those of which our patients tell us they frequently come into contact with.

We should also always be thinking about what we are putting *into* our bodies. The old saying, "you are what you eat" is very appropriate here, and we will talk more about nutrition and what we should and shouldn't be eating in chapter 7.

For this chapter, we thought it prudent to talk about the changing agricultural landscape of the UK. In comparison with the rest of the world, we are a tiny island. Land is at a premium, and farming is moving further away from arable crops and moving more towards livestock. Our passion for eating and exporting meat is on the rise, and farming methods have had to adapt to feed this demand. In recent years, we have bred our livestock to either produce more milk, or to be heavier and give us more meat. But breeding will only get us so far. In order to speed this process up, some farmers may give growth hormones to their animals. In the recent past, our chickens have been farmed in large warehouses, often in cramped conditions. Diseases are spread very easily in this environment, so our chickens are often fed antibiotics and antivirals to help combat this. Growing crops can be a risky business. Not only are you battling the elements —too much rain and they drown, too little rain and they dry out— but there are all those creatures that want to eat those crops as well. The most common way of combating the pest problem is to spray the crops with pesticides.

Where do all those hormones, drugs and pesticides go once they have been given to our animals or sprayed on our crops? The answer is that they tend to stay either on, or *in* the food that we are eating. We are therefore ingesting it. As good as our livers are at removing these substances from our blood, some pesticides can build up in the body and can even cause health problems. Pesticides have also been known to get into our soil and waterways and end up in our drinking water. We recommend that as often as you can, eat organic food, filter your tap water, and wash all your fruit and vegetables thoroughly.

Your body is a natural being and "runs" better if we supply it with natural produce. Be careful of the quantities of e-numbers, caffeine and fake sugars you are consuming. We will talk more about these in chapter 7. One thing we will say on the topic of sugar and caffeine is that they both give you natural highs; our body craves these, which is why they can become so addictive. The problem is that with the highs come the inevitable lows and mood swings. You will remember from earlier that your mood can affect your posture, and your posture can affect the amount of physical stress you place your body under.

Not only are we ingesting chemicals that have no place in our diets, but we are choosing to breathe them in as well. Many of us love our homes smelling fresh and clean. We use air freshener sprays or plug-ins. Unfortunately, the majority of these pump out laboratory-made, synthetic fragrances. We breathe these chemicals in and our bodies have to process them. If you love your air fresheners and cannot be parted from them, look out for organic, natural-scented products. They tend to be in the form of candles or scented reeds. We use organic, scented reeds in our centre, and members of our community often make positive comments on them.

We also come into physical contact with chemicals everyday - have you ever wondered what makes your antibacterial hand washes or wipes antibacterial? Most of these products contain a compound called Triclosan. So if this substance kills bacteria and then it's on your hands, when you touch your eyes or mouth, it can get into your body. Some studies have suggested that using antibacterial products may be contributing to antibiotic resistance, and can even produce hormonal effects.

There is little evidence to show that antibacterials work any better than normal soaps. Your body has its own, very well-developed way of dealing with bacteria and other foreign bodies: it's called your immune system. If we continue killing off bacteria, especially when we are young, our immune systems will struggle to develop and adapt to different strains of bacteria in the future.

As Chiropractors, we believe you are always better off with a better functioning spine and a nervous system that functions well, than one that doesn't.

There was a flu pandemic in 1918, which was labelled one of the most devastating outbreaks ever. It has been estimated that 20-40 million people died worldwide because of it. Over 675,000 Americans lost their lives but interestingly enough it was deemed to be a turning point in the Chiropractic profession. Why? By then, Chiropractic had been around for 23 years and was gathering a dedicated following of patients. It was noted that at the same time, statistically fewer of those patients who were receiving Chiropractic care died from this pandemic than those not receiving care. Here follows some of the statistics from the day:

"In Davenport, Iowa 50 medical doctors cared for 4,953 cases with 274 deaths. Also in Davenport, 150 chiropractors saw 1,635 cases with only one death. In the state of Iowa, medical doctors treated 93,590 patients, with 6,116 deaths, a loss of one patient out of every 15. In the same state, excluding Davenport, 4,735 patients were seen by chiropractors with a loss of only six patients – a loss of one patient out of every 789.

National figures show that 1,142 chiropractors cared for 46,394 for influenza during 1918, with a loss of 54 patients – one out of every

859. In New York City, 950 out of 10,000 cases died with medical methods while 25 out of 10,000 died using drugless methods.

Yes, the medical profession was seeing a majority of the worst of the worst; however, one of the greatest statistics backing chiropractic care comes from the state of Oklahoma. There were 233 cases in which the medical doctors had cared for patients and eventually pronounced them as "lost" or beyond hope… Chiropractors took care of all 233 with only 25 deaths.

Chiropractic's journey into health care took a huge leap forward thanks to its incredible effect on the thousands of Americans during the flu crisis. People came to see first-hand the amazing results that can be obtained with the Chiropractic adjustment. When you get adjusted, you increase immune function. An increase in immune function is important for everything from the cold and runny nose to influenza, cancer, and heart disease. An adjustment will stimulate your immune system to better fight off any illness in your body."

[excerpt from The Flu Epidemic of 1918, England Chiropractic and Nutrition].

We believe that this lends credence to the fact that Chiropractic patients tend to have stronger immune systems and get sick less, great bonus!

Did you know that your skin is the largest organ in your body? Please be careful which deodorants, perfumes and lotions you smother it in or wash it with. Check labels for a substance called Sodium Laureth Sulphate or Sodium Lauryl Sulfate. This is a surfactant which makes things like shampoo, shower gels and toothpastes foam up. This compound has been linked to skin damage and liver toxicity. Look for more natural products without this ingredient.

Medication

Interestingly enough, Wendy's mum is a pharmacist and a life-long believer in Chiropractic care, and she credits her mum for inspiring her chosen career. Wendy often tells the story that when she was growing up, her friends were often given over-the-counter medications. If they had a headache, they took some paracetamol. If they had a tummy ache, they would take some antacids. If they fell over and bruised themselves, aspirin was the drug of choice. Now, you would have thought that Wendy's mum, being a pharmacist, with easy access to all of the above, would have been the first to hand them out when Wendy came home after falling off her skateboard or tumbling out of a tree for the umpteenth time. But no, the advice was always, "Oh well, never mind, dust yourself off, drink plenty of water and you will be fine."

So, why was this? The main reason could have been that every drug you take has a side effect of some sort. The common ones are dry eyes and a dry mouth and an upset stomach. The main reason these drugs make it into our drug stores and pharmacies is that the side effects are outweighed by the positive effects. A good example of this is the painkiller, Ibuprofen. Ibuprofen commonly upsets the lining of your stomach and chronic (long term) use can lead to, in some susceptible users, stomach ulcers. You also can't take it if you are asthmatic or on heart medication, due to the negative interactions these drugs have on each other.

Other medications, such as Co-codamol, can cause constipation, which is why many patients who have been on long term painkillers are not only on antacids for their stomachs but are also on a laxative for their bunged-up bowels. Granted, painkillers are good at blocking pain signals from your body to your brain, but the longer you take them, the more likely you are to end up increasing the dosage or the number of tablets you take. This is because the body gets better at breaking the drug down and becoming immune to it. You then end up taking more drugs, which leads to more side effects, which leads to more drugs to combat *those* side effects —which can then lead to toxic overload.

Statins are yet another commonly-prescribed drug. Statins reduce cholesterol, a fatty substance that lines the arteries and acts as a lubricant allowing your blood to move smoothly along. We all need a certain amount of cholesterol in our bodies to do this, but too *much* narrows and blocks arteries leading to high blood pressure, heart disease and strokes, which is where statins come in. That said, we have had patients who come to see us regularly who are in their 80s, who have a history of high cholesterol, but have chosen not to go on statins as they believe the side effects are not outweighed by the benefits.

A great example of this was one of our patients who at 81 had a cholesterol reading of seven on the lipoprotein analysis test. This blood test checks the level of the fatty substance, cholesterol, in the blood. A good or acceptable reading would be below five mol/L. His GP wanted to prescribe him statins again. But he refused. His reason was that, in his previous experience of the drug, he started to have terrible muscle cramps in his legs. The cramps were so bad that he couldn't sleep, so he was tired and irritable. He stopped taking them and the cramping stopped. This is no surprise, considering that studies have linked statins to muscle cramping and muscle wastage.

Studies indicate that a certain amount of "good cholesterol" in the body is needed for good health (as it is needed for cell walls and steroid production). Interestingly enough, a cholesterol reading of seven was considered normal a few years ago, but because of studies linking a "high" level of cholesterol with disease, pharmaceutical companies recommended this level be reduced to five, resulting in more people falling into the "at risk" category and being recommended statins. It does makes us wonder though about all those patients who weren't prescribed statins before the level was reduced to five. I can't remember mass deaths being reported, can you? Indeed, there is research which now questions just how effective statins really are in preventing strokes, so the days of prescribing them so readily could soon be under review.

Another drug we see a lot of people taking who are suffering with long term pain is antidepressants. Long term pain can really grind you down; it stops you from doing all those things you enjoy, like playing sports, socialising with your family and friends, and functioning well at work. Unfortunately, antidepressants, although helpful in the short term, can be highly addictive, and in our opinion should not be used as a long-term solution. Seek help in a more natural way, whether that is through Chiropractic care and/or brain training techniques such as cognitive behavioural techniques; there is a lot of help out there if you choose to seek it.

A great way of boosting your own happy hormones or endorphins is to exercise. Exercising, especially something that uses your calf muscles, is great, as this stimulates the release of endorphins. We recommend that you exercise three times a week for 30 minutes at a time. Walking is a great form of exercise, being low impact and kinder to the joints of your body. More about exercising in chapter 8.

All this talk about being in pain and taking pain medications reminds us of a lady who came to see us when we were still practicing in our centre on Bolton street. Our practice there was up four flights of stairs and you may be forgiven for thinking that this was a poor location for a Chiropractic centre whose patients with bad backs were being made to walk (and indeed, sometimes, *crawl*) up all those stairs. But we used to say it separated those patients who really wanted to come and see us to improve their health, from those who were less, shall we say, *committed*. Now, this lady didn't walk up the stairs, she was carried up there by her husband. She had hurt her lower back a year earlier, lifting one of her children into their car seat. The pain was intense, and normal painkillers weren't touching it, so this lady was taking a highly addictive form of pain blocker called morphine. Even on morphine, her back pain was so severe that she could no longer walk unaided —and she was only in her early 30s. The morphine was at such a dose that she wasn't herself anymore. She was spending her days in a slightly "spaced out" condition, her relationship with her husband was fractious, and to add to the pressure, they were also wanting to start trying for another baby.

One of the most amazing things was getting to witness this lady, over a period of 8-12 months, change from being in constant pain to less pain, to walking again, to eventually decreasing her morphine dose, and eventually coming off it. She became pain-free and went back to living a normal life. She now runs a highly successful textile business, and has a new baby son. It sounds like a miracle, but if you remove the cause of the pain, which in this case was nerve irritation, the body is very capable of healing itself, it just needs a helping hand to steer it in the right direction at times.

PHYSICAL STRESS AND BEING BORN

Talking of babies leads us nicely onto the third category of stress which is, "physical." We get asked all the time, "how old is the youngest person that you see here?" Most are astonished when we tell them "a couple of weeks old." Just in case you were wondering, our eldest patient is 93 years of age and counting. But back to babies. There is a popular theory that the most physically stressful thing you will ever go through in your life is being born. Think about it. A baby's head, which is about the size of a small honeydew melon, is passing through an area that is normally the size of an orange. The pressure on the head and shoulders is enormous. Now, think about what happens to the baby if a little help is needed; for example, in the form of forceps around the head. The head can be rotated excessively until the shoulders come through, and the baby is born. Can you imagine the effect this has on those little neck bones and the nerves that they protect? This is also the case when forceps are not an option and a Ventouse delivery is chosen (a method where the baby is delivered with the assistance of a vacuum extraction device).

Perhaps an emergency caesarean section is needed. At this point, the baby will already be in the birth canal. A surgical slit is made at the bikini line, and the surgeon reaches in and grabs whatever body part they can get hold of: head, shoulder, or hip —and then the baby is pulled and squeezed out through this narrow gap. These body parts can be easily injured. So the process of being born, even at the best of times, can be quite traumatic and can put the body through a great deal of physical stress.

Babies are, thankfully, very resilient and they generally do recover fairly quickly, although there are times when residual effects from the birthing process remain, causing spinal misalignments. We find this often manifests in babies as colic. They may also be poor sleepers.

A story which springs to mind is that of a couple who had recently had a baby. This baby had been born via emergency Caesarean section, as the little boy had become distressed during labour trying to exit the birth canal, resulting in a very unhappy baby.

He suffered with dreadful colic and the parents were beside themselves with worry and lack of sleep due to his non-stop crying. They had tried the G.P. but nothing seemed to be working and they knew they couldn't continue as they were. The parents brought their son to see us, so we felt along the baby's spine and located a particularly jammed joint in the neck which we believed to be irritating a nerve resulting in pain or discomfort, hence the constant crying. We worked gently on this area, with fingertip pressure, and over a period of several weeks, the baby began to settle down and sleep. We felt so honoured to have been able to help, and it was wonderful when the mother thanked us for "giving her life back," to this day she still continues to bring her son in for regular check-ups.

When you examine an adult spine from the side, it has three curves. When babies are born, though, they haven't yet developed those curves.

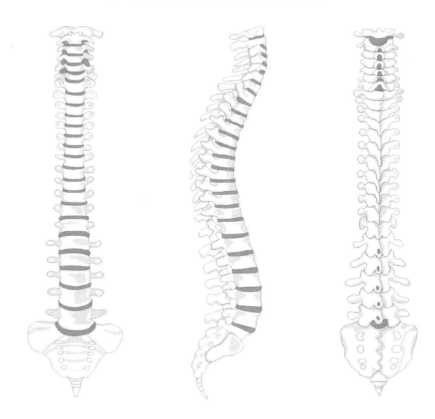

Diagram showing the three curves of the spine: From top to bottom - Cervical, Thoracic and Lumbar.

The cervical (neck) lordotic curve consists of seven vertebrae, and develops when your baby learns to hold their head up. The second curve down is the thoracic, (sometimes referred to as the kyphotic curve), and is made up of 12 vertebrae, where the ribs come out and develops when you learn to sit. The last is the lumbar curve, which is sometimes called the lower lordotic curve, and this comprises five vertebrae, and develops when the baby starts to stand and walk.

All babies are born with their spinal column closely resembling the letter "C." Now, imagine that one of those spinal joints has been pushed out of place during the birthing process. When the baby lies on its back, it is right on the sore part. This will be uncomfortable, and will most likely result in the baby sleeping poorly and crying in discomfort.

Babies who don't crawl for long, as it is uncomfortable for them to be in that position, often skip crawling for walking. This can affect the development of the muscles in the child's mid-back. With these muscles being underdeveloped, this can exacerbate underlying problems, which can lead to symptoms later on in life.

We believe that "baby bouncers", moulded baby seats and "walkers" are not the best for helping babies. Remember, babies are born with a "C" shaped spine. When they begin to sit this places pressure on the lower spinal bones and discs. Babies will naturally choose to stop sitting and change positions to relieve this pressure build-up but find this very hard to do if they are trapped, sitting in a "walker", "bouncer" or moulded seat. These devices keep a baby in a c curve position so the Cervical and Lumbar spines don't have time to develop. Without tummy time a baby cannot strengthen the necessary muscles needed to provide the strength to move e.g. rolling, sitting and crawling – all very important movements. If the baby is forced to sit before physiologically ready the entire weight of the head is placed upon the spine. When the spine and muscles are not fully developed in terms of strength this risks spinal degeneration.

Babies who are allowed to choose to move more naturally would change from this seated position to a crawling one sooner. Babies then develop their low back or lumbar curve with tummy time, creeping and crawling. Tummy time and crawling is very important as it helps to develop nice strong low back muscles to give support to the spine for the next phase, standing and walking.

The great news is that Chiropractic care uses gentle techniques to correct these spinal joint misalignments, allowing babies to become more comfortable. We often see that our infant patients sleep better, have less colic, and can "latch on" better when being breastfed.

Fast forward a few months and babies are growing up, crawling, standing, walking, running, and falling over. In fact, by the age of five, it is estimated that a child will have fallen hundreds of times —of which many are significant and could cause joint immobility. It's important to get children checked regularly, not only to make sure that their three spinal curves are developing as they should, but also to try and prevent any knocks and bumps sustained during play leading to problems later on in life.

We have lost count of the number of times our patients have said, "I wish I had known about Chiropractic care years ago, I needn't have been putting up with these problems for so long!" How amazing would it feel if you had had Chiropractic all your life, from birth?

Just one of the things that we love about what we do on a daily basis is helping families stay happy and truly well; herein lies a tale of what we see played out over and over again in our centre. Normally, it is the Mum that comes to see us first. Then Mum brings her husband in with her for her Verbal Report of our Findings (where she discovers exactly what is causing her symptoms, how long it will take her to get better and how much it will cost.) Once Mum is on the mend and has been a successful "guinea pig" for the family, the husband comes in for help. Once both parents are on the mend, then the little ones start to come and see us. It's very satisfying for us to see those little ones, that we first saw when they were either babies or in nursery, who are now either in secondary school or off to University. We love seeing families like these, enjoying living life to its fullest.

Whiplash Type Injuries

Sometimes, situations occur that you didn't plan for or foresee. We are of course talking about those bad trips and falls, sporting injuries, or knocks and bumps sustained in traffic jams when the driver behind goes into the back of you. Or that driver in front of you that could have gone at that roundabout but decided not to, and you bump into the back of them. Sound familiar? We see a lot of these "whiplash" type injuries.

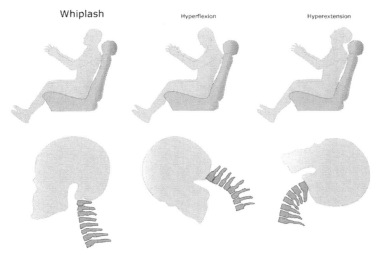

Whiplash   Hyperflexion   Hyperextension

Diagram showing what happens to the neck during a front-on collision.

Seen from the side, looking towards the left, the neck curve should look like the letter "C." We have sadly seen many X-rays where this curve has been forced to straighten. This occurs when the head and neck are suddenly forced backwards and then forwards so quickly with such extreme stress that the supporting musculature is unable to protect the neck. This is commonly seen on the X-rays of those who have been in car accidents, but we also see it in assault cases, in people who play rugby and football and in falls. In fact, we see it whenever people have taken part in high impact injuries involving extreme acceleration/deceleration. This can not only affect your neck but can also affect your lower back as well. The "C" curves are there to absorb axial compression and act as a shock absorber when you walk. Imagine where pressure points start to build up in your spine if you now have a straightened curve. Pressure builds up throughout and left to its own devices, this can worsen with time, leading to wear and tear and even arthritis. Don't worry, we have seen thousands of these type of injuries over the years and the vast majority improve with Chiropractic care. But you don't need to have had a major car accident, fallen off your bike, or even had a traumatic birth to develop misalignments in your spine and extremities.

The majority of people who come to see us have physical stresses brought on by micro-traumas from small trips up the stairs, sprained ankles, poor working conditions, ergonomics and bad posture which have accumulated over time. The body is fantastic at adapting to change, but problems and pain become more noticeable when the body runs out of compensatory options. This is why you may feel that you have recovered from a slip or fall only to suffer symptoms later -sometimes even *years* down the line.

Don't worry though —it's never too late to do something about it. Don't let stress stop you from doing the things you and your family love to do. If you are sitting there, reading this book and thinking that you can't afford manual, holistic therapies such as Chiropractic care, then think about what life would be like if you didn't take action now.

Many people who come to see us are self-employed hairdressers, landscapers, roofers, builders, farriers, and business owners. One particular gentleman who regularly comes to see us, is a landscaper and mountain bike fanatic.

He regularly comes off his dual-suspension mountain bike, but it's his years and years of wheel-barrowing soil, digging up trees, planting, laying down paving slabs and rolling turf that has, over time caused the wear and tear in his spine. He doesn't earn a huge salary but he knows if he doesn't have regular spinal checks ups, like you would for your teeth, that he could pick up more injuries which would mean he couldn't work. If he can't work, he doesn't earn money, and if he doesn't earn money then he can't afford to feed his family. So, he sets aside some of his wage every month so that he can afford Chiropractic care, because he can't afford *not* to have it. It's a big part of his lifestyle and it could be part of yours, too, if you choose it.

In our Centre (as with many others), we make Chiropractic care as affordable as possible. We are respectful of the time you spend with us, with our team working as efficiently as possible without compromising patient care. Chiropractic care is not only effective in improving the functions of the joints of your body (shoulders, elbows, wrists, hips, knees and feet), but we have seen it help headaches, IBS, jaw problems, ringing in the ears, poor balance, bed-wetting, and it offers a host of other health benefits other than just treating back and neck pains.

Another great way of releasing stress is by having therapeutic or sports massage. Massage helps remove muscle knots and reduce tension. Combining massage with Chiropractic care means you get the best of both worlds, and this can be more effective than just having massage or Chiropractic care on its own.

Chapter summary:

Stress can come from physical, emotional, and/or chemical sources. It's helpful to have a night time routine to reduce your stress levels and thus aid more restful sleep. Be mindful of what you put in and on your body as chemicals may be present. The process of being born can cause misalignments which can manifest later in life if not addressed early. The same is true for whiplash and whiplash-type injuries.

CHAPTER 4:
POSTURE PERFECT

We have touched on this previously, but it's worth mentioning again. The majority of people we see have suffered from an accumulation of micro-traumas over years which have led to their symptoms. One of the major contributory factors is poor posture.

In this chapter, we will be covering what poor posture is, from poor sitting/driving posture, to standing and sleeping positions, and the hints and tips we give our patients to help combat incorrect posture.

The average person will spend 32 years of their life sitting. This could be sitting at home in front of the television, sitting at a desk in work and/or driving to and from work. Did you know that you put more pressure on your lower back when you sit compared to when you stand? Furthermore, if it's true that you are spending 32 years sitting, then we are sure you will agree that it's a great idea to learn how to do it better.

The first thing to do is to make sure that what you are sitting on is adequately supporting you. When sitting on the couch at home, check to make sure it's not too soft and squidgy, forcing you into a slouched position.

When choosing a work office chair, choose one with fully adjustable arm rests and one where you can adjust the height, the angle of the seat, the back rest, and one which has a lumbar support. Only use a foot rest if your feet don't touch the floor. The back rest should be high enough to rest the back of your shoulder blades against, as well as the back of your head.

Check your car seat, make sure it is fairly flat and isn't a "bucket" style seat that slopes upwards at the sides. When you sit in a "bucket" seat it creates a "C" shaped spine (a slumped position) as opposed to an optimally-shaped spine. Check your car seat to see if it has a lumbar support built in, and that it's the right size and height for you.

When sitting in your car, angle the back rest backwards to just off 90 degrees, your bottom should be against the back of the chair and the lumbar support should fill the small of your back. If this isn't the case, deflate or remove the lumbar support and make your own using a loosely rolled-up hand towel and place this into the small of your back instead. Over-pumped, or incorrectly located lumbar supports in cars can be the cause and not the cure of your back problems.

Now that you have the perfect sitting equipment, before you sit down, check to make sure you have nothing in your back pockets. Sitting on something like a mobile phone or a slim wallet will cause the pelvis to be lifted on one side and to become uneven. This places great stress on your lower back and pelvic bones which accumulates with time and can cause low back problems.

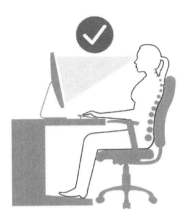 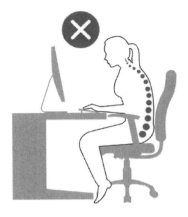

Diagram showing correct sitting posture and what happens to your spine when sitting incorrectly.

The rules of thumb when it comes to a great seated posture are:

- Sit right back into the seat with your bottom against the back of the seat with the back rest angled backwards so that it's just off 90 degrees.

- Use a lumbar support or a small, rolled-up towel and place above your bottom into the curve of your lower back.

- Lower the seat so that your feet rest flat on the ground (or use a foot rest if the desk is too high), hip distance apart, and ensure that your bottom and hips sit higher than your knees. If you cannot angle your seat, then sit on an inflatable seat wedge.

- Lastly and most importantly, never sit with your legs, ankles or knees crossed. Why? Try this out now, wherever you are sitting. Place both feet on the ground. Then sit on your hands. Now cross one leg over the other and feel how one buttock feels slightly heavier than the other. Swap legs and your weight distribution changes again. Over time, this uneven distribution of your body weight through your pelvic bones can cause lower back and hip problems in the future, and it doesn't help the blood circulation in your legs, either. So, if you take only one thing away from this chapter, it should be to remember to, "sit with your ankles or knees uncrossed!"

So now, you are sitting upright but your television is off to one side which means you have to twist slightly to see it. Make sure that what you are watching is straight ahead of you. This also goes for the computer you are using.

The general rule of thumb for setting up your work station is this: Firstly, correct your sitting posture, then pull yourself towards your desk, tuck your arms into your sides and bend your elbows to 90 degrees. Your desk should be at elbow height. Keeping your elbows tucked into your body, move your forearm in an arc from your belly button outwards. Both your keyboard and mouse should live within this arc. As soon as you have to reach or stretch for them, gravity will press down on your arms, causing them to become heavier, which in turn places additional strain on the muscles of your neck and shoulders. Can we ask you a question? Do you ever get a burning sensation behind your neck and between your shoulder blades after a long day sat behind the computer? Did you know that what you are actually experiencing is muscle fatigue? It's also a sure sign that you are either not changing your body position every 30-40 minutes and/or that your work station isn't set up correctly for you.

If you are working with a PC make sure your eyes are level with the top of the screen. If you are using a tablet or laptop, then connect a separate keyboard to it and raise the screen to eye level. This keeps your head, which weighs approximately ten pounds, balancing nicely on the seven little vertebrae that constitute the cervical spine or neck. Remember that for every inch your chin moves forwards, gravity pushes down and adds an additional pound of weight to your head, placing undue stress on both your neck and mid back.

A good standing posture begins with both feet on the ground, spaced hip distance apart. Don't be a "hippy!" By this, we mean don't stand leaning on one leg, popping out the hip, rather, you want to distribute your body weight evenly between both feet. Stand up tall, shoulders and chin back, and keep the knees soft and slightly bent, don't "lock" them out backwards as this causes your pelvis to slump forward, placing stress on your lower back.

We check your posture regularly in the centre, but you can ask someone to check this for you at home, or you can stand side-on next to a full-length mirror. Draw an imaginary line down the side of your body. The line should start from the centre of your ear, pass downwards through the centre of your upper arm, down through the centre of your hip joints, sit just behind the knee cap and end up passing down through the centre of a bone in your foot called the fifth metatarsal head (base of your fifth toe).

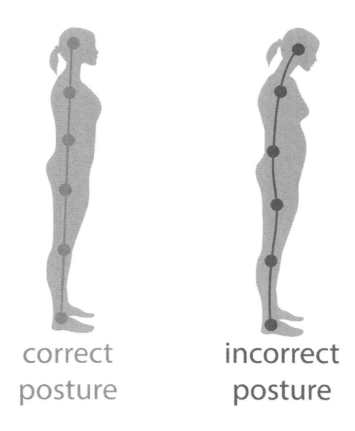

correct posture   incorrect posture

Diagram showing correct standing posture: all points should

be in a straight line.

Now stand with your back to the person who is checking you and ask them to draw imaginary horizontal lines across your body. Are the tips of your ears the same height? Are the tops of your shoulders the same height? Are the tops of your iliac crests the same height? Are your left and right bottom and knee creases the same height? Are you perfect, or, like the vast majority of people who seek our help, a little off and in need of rebalancing?

When standing, can someone place three fingers under the arches of your feet? If they cannot, this means that the arches of your feet could be flat causing the feet to roll inwards. When this happens, your knees move inwards towards each other and you appear to be more "knock-kneed." With your knees and feet rolling inwards, stress is placed not only on your feet and knees but also on your hip joints, pelvis and lower back. If you start to develop mechanical lower back problems, over time, this stress can work its way upwards towards the neck and shoulders and can result in neck pain and headaches amongst other symptoms.

Have you ever noticed that you keep pulling the hem down on one side of your trousers, or that you wear the soles and heels of your shoes unevenly? These are all signs of faulty foot mechanics. When we see this happening in the very young, we teach them exercises to strengthen the arches of their feet and to stretch out their leg muscles but once you've had a fair few birthdays, this problem becomes harder to change as the joints in your feet become more set in their ways. In this case, orthotics can be customised and placed into your shoes, like an innersole, to support your fallen arches, rebalance your body's weight distribution through your feet, and correct your faulty foot mechanics.

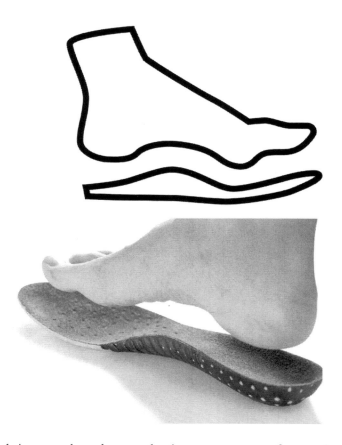

Both images show how orthotics support your foot arches.

As with most things in this world, there are good and not-so-good variations of the same product, and it's no different with orthotics. So, what should you be looking out for? The first thing is to make sure that your feet are checked whilst you are standing (weight-bearing) and walking. The traditional method was to take a plaster cast of your foot whilst you were sitting (non-weight-bearing).Unfortunately, this often gave inaccurate measurements as the shape and function of your foot change when bearing your weight to being non-weight-bearing, thus making those orthotics less effective.

Other more modern techniques include filming your feet whilst you stand and walk, but this is heavily reliant on the practitioner's interpretation to get an accurate result.

The latest, up-to-date method is to use a pressure pad consisting of thousands of tiny sensors, which, when stood on, accurately measure your body's weight distribution through your feet whilst standing still, and whilst you are walking. This information, combined with a physical examination of your feet, is then fed directly to a laptop. We are fortunate to have this system in-house, and it records the information in such a way that you can see, by the use of a colour index, what is happening. We still find it truly fascinating to experience.

We would never feel comfortable recommending something that we ourselves haven't benefited from directly. Let us tell you a story. A few years back, Wendy was climbing a high ropes course with her niece, not far from Blackburn. Pretending to be monkeys swinging through the African jungle, climbing rope ladders and jumping into cargo nets was all great fun until Wendy ascended to the highest point of the course —a rope bridge. Ducking and then twisting under one of the supporting guide ropes, she felt a soft "pop" and a sharp pain come from within her left knee. Weeks of combined Chiropractic and Massage care to rehabilitate her strained ACL ligament followed. The pain went and the function returned, but Wendy was left with what she felt was a slight weak spot in her left knee which, if she were to bend and twist, would flare up once again.

She decided to have her feet scanned here in our Centre, and bespoke orthotics were made. This was when Wendy personally discovered the benefits of orthotics. It felt like she had found the last piece of the jigsaw that was required for her left knee to heal. Wendy now has her prescription moulded into her work sandals as well as removable versions for her other shoes and trainers. One of the most important things to look out for when researching what type of bespoke orthotics you need, as opposed to "off-the-peg" shop-bought versions, is their thickness. Ideally you want them to be only 2-3mm thick as this means that they can fit easily into most shoes. They need to be neither too hard nor too soft, so they are comfortable to wear. It's important to note that if the orthotics are *too* soft, they don't support your feet adequately enough when you are standing and walking as they "give" too easily. If they are too hard, then they can feel restrictive when you walk and place pressure on the joints of your feet. You can choose "ready-to-wear" and "off-the-peg" orthotics from many large sports and pharmaceutical retailers, and they do offer some support for your feet, but they will never be as good as bespoke products.

Have you ever given much thought to your sleeping posture? It might surprise you to know that we spend approximately a third of our lives in bed, so it's actually very important. How old are your pillows and mattress? Eight to ten years is the natural life of a mattress and if yours is about that or older, you should look at replacing it. The support it used to give you will no longer be there. Look to spend the most you possibly can on both your mattress and your pillows, and invest wisely. At the time of print, we would advise that you spend at least £600 on a mattress, choosing one with the highest number of pocket springs as possible.

Are you a person who prefers to sleep on their front? Then stop! Lying on your front causes your lower back to over-arch and means you then have to place your head to one side to enable you to breathe. This places a huge strain on your neck, night after night, and often results in neck, shoulder and arm pain. So stop it! If you lie on your back or on your side, you still need to be mindful that your head and neck are in a neutral position and are well-supported. When sleeping on your side place a pillow between your knees.

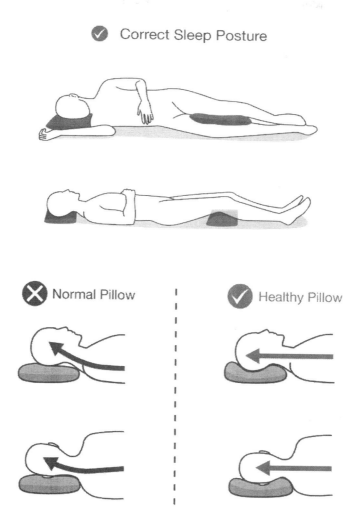

The two diagrams above show correct sleeping posture: where and how to place your pillows to ensure you have a good night's sleep.

Choose your pillow carefully. We tend to advise sleeping on a shaped pillow made of high-density memory foam, which has a raised portion that fits snugly into the space between your shoulder and the side of your neck, whilst your head rests on the lower portion. This ensures that both your head and neck are well-supported whilst you sleep.

Not all memory foam pillows and mattresses are the same, and the rule of "buy cheap, pay twice," can often be applied.

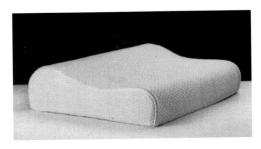

The image above is of a memory foam, shaped neck pillow.

If you sleep mainly on your back, then one traditionally-shaped pillow is usually enough to support the head, but a pillow placed under the knees is helpful too. If you are a 'side sleeper' then we advise the use of a shaped pillow, as this helps you keep your neck in line with your body. Before you buy, we recommend asking a professional to measure you up for the correct sized pillow.

If we had a pound for every time someone asked us to recommend a mattress, or if we could design one that suited everyone, then we would be very wealthy indeed! The truth of the matter is that we are all different shapes, sizes and weights, and so a mattress that suits us may not suit you or your sleeping partner.

We have known couples who have bought their own single beds and pushed them together, rather than having one partner sleeping in their ideal bed whilst the other suffers and experiences poor sleep.

There are some things to consider when sourcing your perfect mattress. The main rule is to lie on (how you would usually lie in bed) and test each mattress you are considering. If you invest the most you can at the time, you won't regret it.

When deciding which ones to test first, go for the medium-to-firm mattress in the range; the more pocket springs, the better. Also lie for ten minutes on your side and ten minutes on your back with your own pillow. Your body needs to maintain that neutral position, with the natural curves of your spine being supported. You are looking for that "aaaaaaah, that feels really comfy" feeling. Not particularly scientific, we realise, but you will "know when you know."

Double check this feeling with a little test. Lying on your back, slide the back of your hand under the small of your back, at about belt level. If you have to "dig" to get under there, then the mattress is too soft. If it "slides" in and out too easily, then it's too hard (yes, a hard mattress isn't necessarily a good mattress), but if it "slots" in, then it's perfect for you. Make sure your bed buddy does the same test with you whilst you are both lying on the mattress. Fingers crossed it suits them too, otherwise single mattresses could be the way forward for you both!

Chapter summary:

We spend roughly 32 years of our lives sitting. It's important to sit correctly in work, in the car, and at home. Remember not to cross your legs or put things in your back pocket and sit on them. Bespoke orthotics can help correct faulty foot mechanics and improve posture. Invest in a good mattress and pillow and try not to sleep on your front as this places stress on your spine.

CHAPTER 5:
X-RAYS

As Chiropractors, we love to look at X-rays. We can gain a lot of information about a patient this way.

Our impression is that the medical profession in general appears to be moving away from X-rays and more towards MRIs, which we will touch on later. We believe, though, that by not x-raying a patient, both they and their practitioner are missing out on a lot of really useful information.

The reason we believe the medical profession is moving away from X-rays is that they are perhaps not using them effectively. Firstly, hospital radiographers tend to take X-rays with the patient in a non-weight-bearing position, i.e. they tend to be lying down. Chiropractors like to take X-rays of the patient standing and thus weight-bearing. Gravity does not have the same effect on the body when you are non-weight-bearing. How much of our lives do we spend lying down? Therefore, how accurate a reflection can these lying down X-rays truly be?

Traditionally, X-rays are taken to rule out sinister causes of pain, such as cancer and other life-threatening conditions in or around the affected joint. Often, if the X-rays have nothing dangerous on them then a report from a radiologist will come back as "normal." This is true from their point of view, if nothing classed as a life-threatening condition was detected. However, this does leave the patient baffled and frustrated wondering what IS causing their symptoms. Indeed, some start to wonder whether they are imagining things. When we were studying at Chiropractic college we had the pleasure of observing a top radiologist at a local hospital.

The number of X-rays we saw him read in a short space of time was truly amazing but what was also astonishing was the number of X-rays that he examined and said, "that's normal," and "*that's* normal." It was astonishing because from a Chiropractic perspective, these X-rays were *not* normal. There were spines that should have been straight when viewed from the front; yet were "S" in shape, displaying scoliosis.

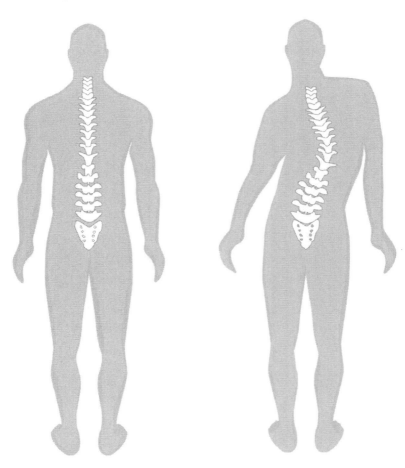

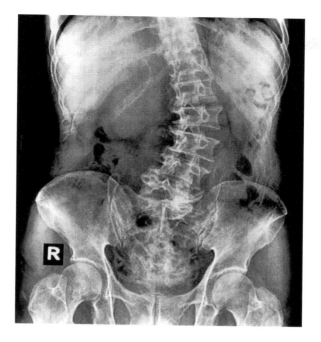

The first diagram shows what an ideal spine should look like compared to one with a scoliosis, and the posture adopted by those who suffer from it. The image above shows what this looks like on an X-ray taken front on.

As you can see from the above pictures, scoliosis is NOT normal. Indeed, a scoliosis can irritate the nerves exiting the spine, resulting in pain and discomfort. From a medical perspective, this can be considered "normal" (when not severe) as it's not cancer, nor is it life-threatening. Mild scoliosis is not believed to cause pain and therefore is not considered significant enough or severe enough to even mention. Yet from a Chiropractic perspective, scoliosis can adversely affect the way the nervous system functions and can result in pain and dysfunction, or in other words, dis-ease within the body.

When Chiropractors examine X-rays, we look at the

alignment of the spine because we know that any vertebrae that is even slightly out of alignment, that isn't quite sat right, can affect the way the nervous system functions, which can lead to a variety of other symptoms.

What can also be confusing at times is that the changes seen on X-rays tend to be described differently between the medical profession and the Chiropractic profession. We have seen reports come back as "normal," yet if we had viewed them we would have noted degenerative changes present at several levels in the spine with some disc wear and bony spurs being present. For the Chiropractor, it is vital to know about these changes as it can affect the areas they adjust and the techniques they choose to use. When the Chiropractor shows you your X-ray and points these changes out to you, then you can quite clearly see them and know what's causing your symptoms. You can see there is a reason you are having problems there. The medical profession in general don't tend to mention degenerative changes on a report unless they are present above a certain level. They do not believe that changes are significant until a certain level of severity has been reached. Chiropractors, however, do believe that any degenerative changes present are *always* significant.

Let's start with explaining what we, as Chiropractors, are looking for on a neck X-ray. On a neck X-ray the curve that should be present plays a vital role in how the spine and nervous system function.

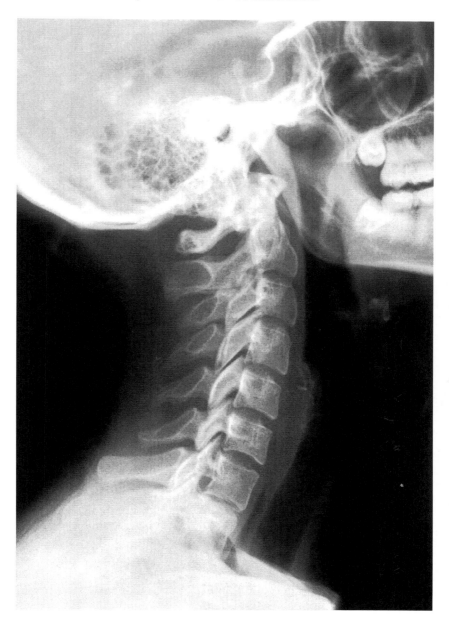

Image of a neck x-ray taken from the side.

When the neck is viewed side on – the spinal column should form a "C" curve. This curve distributes the weight of the head through the spine and into the legs and acts as a shock absorber. Often, particularly after trauma such as car accidents and falls, there can be a straightening of the curve in the neck and a resultant loss of its shock-absorbing capabilities. This results in excessive weight going through the discs and vertebrae of the neck particularly, which accelerates the degenerative process and places added pressure on the nervous system. One of the aims of Chiropractic care is to help restore the normal curve of the neck, which will help take the pressure off the discs and vertebrae and subsequently the nervous system, enabling the body to heal itself.

Some people believe X-rays can be harmful because of the radiation received when exposed to them. We would like to dispel this myth. Firstly, the radiation involved is extremely low.

Put into context, when we go on holiday, we often fly to far away destinations such as the Middle East and America, or those countries closer to us in Europe such as France or Spain. Every time we take a flight, we will be radiated. We may not realise it, but this is because we are flying high above the cloud cover. The stratosphere does protect us from some of the cosmic and solar radiation in the sky but we lose this protection when flying high. The amount of radiation received on a return flight to Spain plus the amount you receive sun bathing on its beaches is more than having a chest X-ray. Now, think about how often pilots and cabin crew fly. These workers are being radiated all the time and their job is not classified as dangerous. Additionally, think about all those celebrities and those on business that fly frequently around the world, either pregnant or with young children. You see newspaper and magazine articles with them sunning themselves in the Maldives one week and skiing in Aspen the next. Very few people think of flying as dangerous as far as radiation is concerned, so why would X-rays be considered a risk?

Additionally, there are certain parts of the UK that have relatively high, naturally occurring radiation levels. Edinburgh is one such area as it is built on granite and when uranium decays in granite it emits radon. Cornwall is another such area, rich in granite and environmental radon, yet these areas are not classified as dangerous places to live.

X-Ray dosage is measured in sieverts (Sv) One sievert is a very large and uncommon dose so sieverts is talked about more as millisieverts (thousandths of a sievert) The UK average annual radiation dose is currently 2.7mSv. This is made up from 5 different sources and nearly half (48%) comes from radioactive radon gas from the ground with the remaining coming from: medical radiation (16%), terrestrial gamma radiation (13%), cosmic radiation (12%), and intakes of radionuclides excluding radon (11%).

Ionising radiation can be found in our soils, water, air and food because it occurs naturally.

Source of Exposure :	Dose:
Dental x-ray	0.005 mSv
100g of Brazil nuts	0.01 mSv
Chest x-ray	0.014 mSv
Transatlantic flight	0.08 mSv
Nuclear power station worker average annual occupational exposure (2010)	0.18 mSv
UK annual average radon dose	1.3 mSv

CT scan of the head	1.4 mSv
UK average annual radiation dose	2.7 mSv
USA average annual radiation dose	6.2 mSv
CT scan of the chest	6.6 mSv
Average annual radon dose to people in Cornwall	6.9 mSv
CT scan of the whole spine	10 mSv
Annual exposure limit for nuclear industry employees	20 mSv
Level at which changes in blood cells can be readily observed	100 mSv
Acute radiation effects including nausea and a reduction in white blood cell count	1000 mSv
Dose of radiation which would kill about half of those receiving it in a month	5000 mSv

Table showing different sources of radiation and their associated levels.

Having your neck X-rayed is equivalent to the dose you would receive by just walking around outside for one-and-a-half days. As you can see from the above, X-rays are low in radiation when compared to other sources, and the benefits really do outweigh the risks.

As technology improves, there seems to be a shift away from cost-effective digital X-rays towards expensive MRIs (Magnetic Resonance Imaging), leading some people to believe that X-rays are now defunct. Let's not beat around the bush, MRIs are expensive. The cost of the equipment runs into hundreds of thousands of pounds and having an MRI scan takes approximately 20 minutes. You may also be in a closed tube-shaped unit, having to stay very still whilst the machine makes some noise. I have known people who have asked to have the procedure stopped because they have felt so claustrophobic. There are, thankfully, more and more open units coming onto the market so claustrophobia is becoming less of a problem.

Comparatively an X-ray takes seconds, the equipment costs tens of thousands of pounds as opposed to hundreds of thousands of pounds and the machine itself is easier and cheaper to maintain. So we do believe X-rays are advantageous when looking at cost and time.

MRIs do produce images where not only the joint but also the disc, the muscles, tendons and ligaments can be visualised. X-rays show bone and disc spaces but not tendons and ligaments —unless they have been calcified. From a Chiropractic perspective, one of the best ways of viewing alignment, which is vitally important to the way the body functions, is by visualising it on an X-ray as opposed to an MRI.

On an MRI, most people will be shown to have a disc bulge or two, where the disc has bulged out of alignment with the spine and which now may be irritating the nerve. Therefore, it come as no surprise to us when an MRI report comes back saying a disc bulge is present. More often than not, though, that disc bulge is NOT symptomatic at that time but it is assumed by most to be the cause of the pain. This is what we call a false positive. There are also times when that disc bulge *is* symptomatic and is the cause of pain. At this stage, an operation may be recommended by a consultant, particularly if consulted privately, to remove part of the disc in an attempt to reduce the symptoms. We have seen many people over the years where this has occurred, who have decided to seek alternative care and after a course of Chiropractic, more often than not, the operation has not been required.

A few years ago, a patient consulted us complaining of extreme lower back pain and raging leg symptoms. She could barely walk -she was limping along, and couldn't really drive as she could only "sit on one butt cheek," and was told that she should stop her horse riding. This was something she had done for approximately 30 years. An MRI scan had revealed a disc bulge irritating the sciatic nerve going into the leg, resulting in the extreme pain she was experiencing. A neurosurgeon had recommended a lower back operation but the patient was not keen to have it and had come to see us because one of her friends had seen us for a similar complaint in the past and had obtained great results. After several months and many adjustments to the spine to relieve the pressure on the nervous system as a whole, the lady was able to go back to horse riding, walk without a limp and drive without being a danger to herself and others on the road. Additionally, her job involved being a carer for her Gran. She had struggled to do this but was now able to once again. This lady still comes to see us regularly to maintain the progress she has made. It is wonderful that she has her life back, and that choosing to have her condition managed this way gave her options other than surgery.

Disc bulges are extremely common and occur when the joints above and below the disc become stuck. The disc itself does not have a direct blood or nutrient supply. It receives its nutrients through the correct movement of the bones above and below it. When the vertebrae above and below the disc are moving, there is lots of fluid gushing into the disc, which acts like a wet sponge. When you compress it, it expands back again. When the vertebrae above and below a disc become jammed, there is a loss of movement and therefore a loss of fluid being released into the disc. The disc then becomes like a *dry* sponge. When you put pressure on it, it gives, causing the disc to wear and bulge.

We believe that this was exactly what happened to a male we saw in his early 40s. He was a teaching assistant suffering from severe neck pain which was causing further sharp pain that was then travelling down into his right arm. His pain was so severe that he could not hold his head up straight and had to tilt it to one side. He could not work, but neither could he afford to stay at home; a few months earlier, he had been forced to declare bankruptcy, the stress of which, we believe, had contributed to his symptoms.

After an examination and X-rays we believed this patient was suffering from a disc bulge in the base of the neck, which was then irritating the nerve and referring pain into his arm. We recommended several months of intensive care, to which the gentleman was unsure he would be able to commit to (due to his bankruptcy). However, he knew he just had to get back to work as he could not live off statutory sick pay, and he begged and borrowed money from his friends to be able to pay for the treatment. Initially, progress was slow, as the disc bulge was so acute and so inflamed, but after completing the recommended course of care, the gentleman was able to return to work. He could hold his head up straight, and the lower back niggles he had been suffering with as well as the severe, sharp neck and arm pain, were gone. He felt like he'd got his life back and the operation on his neck, carrying a risk of paralysis, was negated. He could not have been more grateful.

Surgery to remove part of the disc that has bulged does not restore normal function, as the vertebrae remains stuck and the disc stays "dry." We, as Chiropractors, locate the areas that are stuck, adjust them, and restore normal motion, enabling the movement of fluid back into the disc and the removal of waste products out of it. Chiropractors locate stuck areas on X-rays by examining the alignment of the spine, which cannot be done as easily on an MRI. We therefore believe that X-rays are the gold standard for viewing spinal and joint alignment.

There are very few people who cannot be X-rayed for medical reasons, yet there are many people who cannot have MRIs. People with pacemakers and certain metal joint replacements, for example, cannot have one, because of the extreme magnetism of how an MRI unit works.

Interestingly, although X-rays do show bone, a loss of bone density is only visible on an X-ray once the bone has lost a significant amount of mass. Indeed, figures state this to be anything between 30-50%. However, as practitioners who adjust bones daily, we ensure that those who consult us are asked pertinent questions about smoking, alcohol intake, corticosteroid use and even anorexia, as these can all cause a loss of bone density. We take all these factors into consideration prior to adjusting the bones of your body.

Chapter summary:

Chiropractors utilise X-rays to assess alignment and view degenerative changes. Any and all changes visualised on an X-ray are significant to a Chiropractor. X-rays are low in radiation and are very cost effective. Disc bulges are commonly seen on MRIs, whether or not they are the cause of a patient's symptoms.

CHAPTER 6:
HERE COMES THE SCIENCE BIT / THE HEALING PROCESS TAKES TIME

In this chapter, we will cover a little bit more about the anatomy and function of the spine. Your spinal column comprises 24 mobile bones, each with a disc in between. On average there are 7 cervical (neck) bones, 12 thoracic bones (where the ribs attach), and 5 lumbar (low back) bones. We say, "on average," as there are individuals out there who may never have had an X-ray, and may well be living with extra ribs, extra vertebrae, fused pairs of vertebrae, or malformed bones which they just don't know about. Most tend to be asymptomatic and with the passing of time their amazing bodies have adapted well to them being there.

Pairs of spinal nerves branch out from the spinal column, in between the spinal bones (vertebrae) and travel out into the body. Nothing happens in your body without a nerve signal passing from the brain, down the spinal cord and out through these nerves.

Over time, due to modern day living and the knocks and bumps that life brings, these joints can become stuck. When this happens, they become sore, and the resultant swelling of the surrounding tissues can cause the nerves to become pinched. Pinched nerves can not only become painful but can also adversely affect the organs and tissues they supply, causing dis-ease within the body.

We have had the opportunity to examine and report on thousands of X-rays. We love looking at X-rays. Every person is different and sometimes you will see things you weren't expecting.

One day, a gentleman in his 70s attended the centre complaining of lower back pain and leg symptoms. There was nothing unusual that stood out in his case history, or in the physical examination that we performed, but due to his age and signs of neurological deficit, and the fact he had previously smoked, we undertook a Lumbar spine X-ray prior to commencing care. At this time, we did not have our own digital X-ray machine, and so we used an out-patients clinic that was approximately thirty minutes drive away. The gentleman in question wasn't keen on going for this X-ray, but we insisted upon it. After several minutes of explaining why an X-ray was necessary, the man agreed to have it taken. When the radiologist came to read the X-ray he noticed a massive AAA (Abdominal Aortic Aneurysm) on both the front and side view. He telephoned us straight away to tell us that our patient must go and see his GP urgently for further tests to determine exactly how large this aneurysm was (an aneurysm is where the walls of the artery weaken and bulge, and if they bulge so much they can burst and result in the patient bleeding to death). The GP was called, the patient was seen that day, and had surgery the same week. It was highly likely that the man in question would have died without this life-saving operation. Additionally, the GP surgery changed its own protocol for all males over the age of 70, ensuring that tests were performed on all to rule out AAA in patients exhibiting similar symptoms. It was a huge relief when this gentleman returned to keep us up-to-date with his case and to thank the centre for referring him.

You may think that the degeneration we see would increase as we age. However, this isn't always the case. We have seen 20-year-olds with spines of 50-year-olds, and vice versa. Degeneration is more closely linked to lifestyle choices than just age or genetics. It tends to be the result of years of poor posture, diet, and chemical and physical stresses. Your state of mind and mood also play significant roles.

Did you know there are more than 200 different types of arthritis? The two most common types we see as Chiropractors are Osteoarthritis (OA) and Rheumatoid arthritis (RA). Osteoarthritis or OA is the more common of the two, and is caused by general wear and tear. It tends to affect the joints of the spine and pelvis, the big toes and thumbs, and the hips and knees. When you see this on an X-ray, especially on a side view, you will notice that the disc spaces between the spinal bones have narrowed and often the presence of bony protuberances or bony spurs can be seen (see diagram below). When a radiologist reads your X-rays they will call these bony spurs either osteophytes, osteophytosis, spondylosis or spondylitis. Different words, but they all mean the same thing: "wear and tear"—or arthritis.

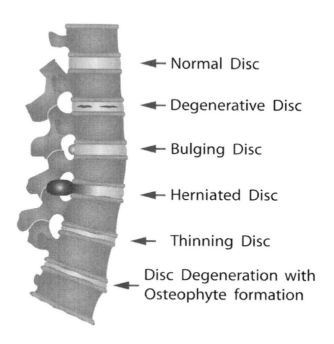

Diagram showing the progression of spinal degeneration: starting from the top and working down.

No matter how long a problem has been there or how bad it is, it's never too late to start looking after yourself. Degeneration can be slowed down, and we have even seen cases where it has been reversed. Did you know that bone remodels itself every ten years? Since bone adapts to the stress being placed upon it, reducing that stress can in some cases reverse the "wear and tear" present. For example, if you have OA in the joints of your lower back, and you have those same joints realigned, reducing the stress placed on them, then the vertebrae can, over time, have an opportunity to remodel.

A gentleman who had been coming to see us for years to help maintain the health of his spine suffered a flare up between appointments. Rather than call us for an adjustment, he decided it was that bad that he had to go to A and E. Once there, he underwent an MRI scan and a disc herniation or bulge was revealed. An operation was recommended and given his MRI results; his spine was fused. This all occurred in a very short time frame and between his monthly appointments. Following on from the surgery, his pain was really no better and so he returned to the centre for a second opinion and for Chiropractic care. We couldn't believe what had happened in between his appointments, and how, over a period of just a few short months, his spine had been fused with two metal rods. An X-ray we subsequently took showed exactly what had been done.

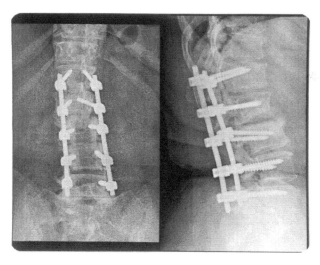

The above image is of a lower back X-ray post spinal fusion surgery. Note the white metal nuts and bolts holding the metal rods in place.

One of the most frustrating things was that we compared an up-to-date x-ray with one we'd taken three years earlier, and found that the wear and disc space shown on this x ray was no worse than it had been 3 years ago! The care we had been delivering had really slowed down the degenerative process, it had not got any worse. Post-op, this patient required another course of care due to the changes brought on as a result of the surgery. The great news was that by the end of this course, he was much more mobile and back to his normal self.

It must be stressed that degeneration is not the cause of your problems, but rather a *symptom* caused by something you have done in the past or are continuing to do in the present. Change this by realigning your body and you can change the situation that you currently find your body in. Are pain and discomfort simply the expected symptoms of ageing; something you just have to put up with? No! It is your body telling you to seek help so it can be changed and improved.

The second most common type of arthritis we see is Rheumatoid arthritis or RA, which is quite different from Osteoarthritis. Whilst osteoarthritis occurs over time, Rheumatoid arthritis is an autoimmune disease. This is when the body malfunctions and starts to "attack" itself. RA is linked to a protein found in white blood cells, called HLA-B27. A blood test can detect the presence of this protein. More often than not, this protein lies dormant until something activates it.

Pregnancy can cause RA to flare up because of hormonal changes, only to then calm down post-partum, and the reverse can also be true. Symptoms of RA include warm, swollen and painful joints, which often worsen with rest. This is why people with RA can often feel worse in the morning and then easier as the day progresses. RA tends to affect both sides of the body, with the joints of the hands and feet being commonly affected. Symptoms also include periods of inflammation followed by periods of remission; it is possible to suffer from both Rheumatoid and Osteoarthritis at the same time.

As Chiropractors, we must know if any of our patients have Rheumatoid arthritis, and actively look for inflammatory periods as this often causes ligament laxity. There is a ligament called the Atlanto-dentoid ligament situated in the upper part of the neck, which stabilises the second cervical vertebrae (C2) inside the spinal column. If this ligament becomes lax (which it can with RA), it can result in the instability of C2. This is why it is important for us to know, so we can modify how we adjust this area. This is also one of the reasons we take an extremely thorough medical case history before we adjust anyone. We would never take a chance with your health or our reputation, ever!

X-rays are amazing, but the one thing they don't show so well are the intervertebral discs, the discs which act as spacers and shock absorbers between the spinal bones. We can see the space that a disc occupies on an x-ray and we can measure the height of the space the disc occupies, but as discs consist mainly of fluid, X-rays pass straight through them, unlike bone, which is more dense.

The discs in the spine are made up of three parts. In the centre sits a ball-bearing-like structure, called the nucleus pulposus. Surrounding the nucleus is a jelly-like matrix, and holding everything together is the tough outer layer called the annulus fibrosis.

Anatomy and physiology of the vertebrae

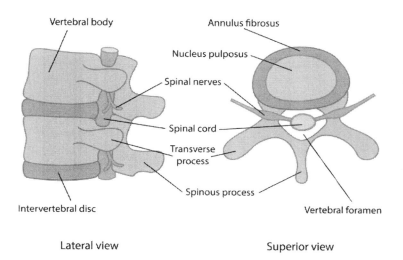

Lateral view   Superior view

The nucleus pulposus allows easy pivoting of the spinal bones which sit above and below it. It's this that gives your spine its global range of movement. This movement is then controlled by the facet joints and the surrounding ligaments and muscles which attach to the spinal bones nearby. The disc also acts as a spacer between the bones, allowing space for the nerves to exit.

With every step you take, small shock waves move upwards from your feet to your knees, to your hips, pelvis and finally into the spine. The jelly-like matrix which surrounds the nucleus pulposus acts like a shock absorber, absorbing some of the impact and protecting the nerves that pass out between each level of the spinal column. As you gain more birthdays, your discs can become dehydrated and you lose height, which can be a reason people "shrink," or get shorter as they age.

There are many times we are told, "I think I have a slipped disc." This isn't technically true. Think of your disc as a small jam doughnut. If you rub the walls of the doughnut enough, you will cause them to become thinner and weaken. Now squeeze the doughnut on one side and watch the jam filling push up against the inside wall of the doughnut. Squeeze harder and the jam will cause the wall to bulge. Squeeze quickly and hard enough and the jam will rupture or herniate through the wall of the doughnut, and escape. This is what can happen to the discs of your spine if your spinal bones are out of alignment, they can rub on the annulus fibrosis (the wall of the doughnut), causing it to weaken. With a weakened wall, all it can take sometimes is for you to simply bend, or twist and lift and the disc can bulge.

So discs can bulge and herniate but they never "slip" out of place. With the spinal nerves exiting so close to the disc, any decrease in the disc's height, due to dehydration or bulging, can cause narrowing of the space where the nerves exit, causing irritation and pain (see diagram below). Ultimately, this can then affect the tissues, muscles and organs that *that* nerve supplies.

Spinal disc herniation

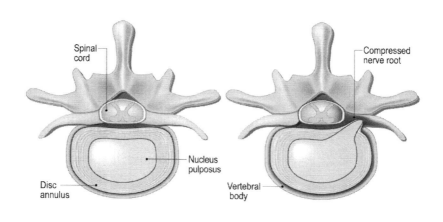

Spinal cord

Compressed nerve root

Nucleus pulposus

Disc annulus

Vertebral body

NORMAL DISC   HERNIATED DISC

Diagram showing disc herniation and how the "jam" can cause a bulge in the wall of the "doughnut" and place pressure on the nerve.

The great news is that Chiropractic care is very effective in helping those with disc problems. One such story we will share here. We saw a gentleman who was in his early thirties when he sought our care. He had to climb up our stairs on his hands and knees and when he reached the top, he couldn't stand up straight. In fact, he was bent over double towards his left. He was ashen with pain. As always, we completed a thorough neurological and orthopaedic examination and we also took a set of Lumbar X-rays. He was in such agony that some of the tests couldn't even be performed! However, his X-ray results showed severe reduction of the last disc space of his spine and that, coupled with absent reflexes in his left foot and ankle, and along with other test results, indicated that he had a disc bulge in the left-hand side of the last disc in his lower back. Over a number of weeks we worked on his spine, enabling the body to heal itself and function better. As the weeks went by and the pain stopped, we got to know him really well. He told us he had been having low back niggles for years before this incident, but being a busy, self-employed, long-distance lorry driver, he had never found the time to get those niggles sorted. If he had sought help when those niggles had first reared their ugly heads, he might never have reached the condition he was in when he first came to us (not being able to walk, sit or drive his truck). It took months of hard work and commitment from the both of us until he could firstly stand up straight, then walk without limping and finally, return to driving. But we got there. We've been friends for over eight years now and we always look forward to catching up and hearing about his travels around Britain and beyond.

Another common question we are asked is, "how long is it going to take for me to feel better?" The answer to this varies depending upon what you have, how long it's been there, and to a certain extent, how old you are. Sadly, on average, the older we get, the slower we heal. Soft tissue injuries take many months to heal and the process can take up to two years. This is one of the reasons we commonly recommend a three-month course of care to begin with. This normally includes gentle, manual adjustments to improve the alignment of the bones (to enable the nervous system to function at its most optimal to allow the body to heal), advice on using ice, nutritional and postural advice, as well as simple stretches and exercises that can be performed at home.

The body takes time to heal, but not all body tissues heal at the same rate. It can take muscles a number of days to four weeks or more, bone, six to twelve weeks, and ligaments many months, even years to heal. So, when we come to design a care plan specifically for you, we will always take into consideration the healing time of the tissues affected. This determines what we decide to do, how we do it and when we decide to do it, thus ensuring maximum benefit to the body.

Few injuries involve just one body tissue. Most injuries involve a combination of bone, nerve, muscle and ligament. For example, if you break a bone in the lower leg (e.g. the tibia), not only does the fracture affect this bone but also the ligaments and tendons which attach near or onto that area. In fact, ligaments only begin to fully recover once you are out of pain. So you may be pain-free, but for the ligaments, the healing process has only just begun.

One particular lady had been having problems with her left knee. As she had private medical insurance she decided that she wanted a surgeon's opinion. The surgeon wanted to clean the joint out, a procedure known as an arthroscopy, which involves shaving off excess bits of bone growth and clearing up the joint by sucking out these bits. We advised the lady to give the body more time to heal as we were working on the knees, but we were still in the infancy of care and we had a long way to go. She decided to proceed with an arthroscopy anyway, and sadly ended up having more pain and less mobility than before. The result was a further arthroscopy and a cortico-steroid injection into both knees. Consequently, this lady had to use sticks to walk and was in considerable pain, not just around the knee but also in the lower part of her back. She returned to us for Chiropractic care, and after having more time to work on her knees and lower back and the body having sufficient time to heal, she is now more mobile than she has been in months. The healing process takes time and cannot be rushed!

Pain can be deceptive. Even when the pain has gone away, you are rarely back to functioning optimally, as this takes much more time. Our advice is to always invest your time and money to not only get yourself out of pain, but to also get your body back to functioning correctly. You may initially think that this involves a fair amount of money and time but the long-term repercussions of not doing this far outweigh the short-term benefits you gain by stopping care.

If you punctured all your car's tyres, you would need to replace them. You need your car to get to work, take the children to school, and so on. You would find the money for the new tyres somehow, even if you couldn't afford it and had to borrow and beg. A car is a necessity for most of us these days. If your washing machine stopped working, you need clean clothes, so you would spend the hundreds of pounds it would cost to replace it, again finding the money from somewhere even if you couldn't afford it. We all think of cars and washing machines as must-have items; we could not live without them. These are all however, tangible, perishable items and can be replaced fairly easily if necessary.

Many people go on holiday once a year, it's a break from the norm and gives you a chance to relax and de-stress and do things you wouldn't usually do. We can spend weeks counting down to a holiday and looking forward to it. We can spend many hundreds of pounds on not just the actual holiday itself but all the other "bits" which go with it, like new clothes, for example. This is all for the enjoyment of a week or two away. Don't get us wrong, holidays are "our thing," and the thing we love to spend our money on, too. However, life is poor if your health is suffering. What good is a week away in the sun when you can't enjoy it because of constant back pain? What good are four new tyres if you can't drive for long periods of time and can't get to work because of neck and arm pain? What good is a new washing machine if you can't bend your knees to get your clothes in and out of it?

In our experience, people spend their money on what they *want* to spend it on. Some choose to head out for a night on the town, thinking nothing of spending a hundred pounds on alcohol, yet they wouldn't spend that same amount on food. Others love to buy clothes and accessories, spending a few hundred pounds on a handbag, but they wouldn't spend that same amount of money on a washing machine as they "couldn't afford it." But what good are fancy clothes when you feel fatigued because of a constant headache or shoulder pain? You only get one spine and nervous system so it's essential to make the most of the one you have. Your body has to last you a lifetime —clothes, cars, and washing machines can be replaced. Missing that yearly holiday so you can invest the money and time needed to improve your health means you get to enjoy the holiday the following year so much more.

Chapter summary:

Degeneration is more lifestyle-dependant than age-dependant. There are over 200 different types of arthritis and most can be managed effectively with appropriate Chiropractic care. Discs cannot "slip" out of place, but can bulge and herniate. The healing process takes time as bone, muscle, ligament and nerve have different healing times. You only get one body, so make the most of the one you have.

CHAPTER 7:
YOU ARE WHAT YOU EAT

Did you know that the human body consists of up to 60 percent water? The average person should be drinking at least two litres of water a day. Now, when we say water we don't mean tea, coffee, carbonated drinks or juices but pure, unadulterated, good old-fashioned water. Keeping hydrated is so important for maintaining good health. Not only does it help keep our body tissues supple and intervertebral discs "plump," but the chemical processes of the body require water in order to work. Water can increase energy levels, reduce certain headaches, help with mental concentration levels, and also aid digestion.

Chronic dehydration is problematic as it can cause a loss of disc height. When the discs narrow, the vertebrae come closer together which can then cause the gap, where the nerves exit the spine in between the bones, to become smaller. The nerve can then become pinched, leading to dysfunction and pain. The nerves from this region travel towards your stomach and diaphragm, and any pressure on the nerves here can starve the organs of vital nerve impulses which can affect a person's ability to take a deep breath, cause acid reflux (heartburn) or indigestion, and, in some cases, stomach ulcers. There is little point in being mindful of what you choose to eat if your body cannot process it well due to stomach issues. Interestingly enough, we have seen patients who have attended our centre solely for their mid back pain, who have had a course of Chiropractic care, and then gone on to experience an improvement in their breathing, heartburn and acid reflux.

How you spend your days will also determine how much water you should be drinking. People who perform manual work need to drink more water and should aim to drink between two to four litres a day. If you are an office worker breathing in dry, air-conditioned air then you will also need a minimum of two litres per day, or six to eight large glasses. If it's a hot day, then you will need to consume even more. Now, we know what you are thinking, especially if you are not used to drinking this volume of water: firstly, how am I going to get all that liquid in, and secondly, won't I be spending half my day visiting the toilet? If you started today by drinking your usual one pint of water to suddenly consuming eight pints then yes, the likelihood is that your kidneys, which are not used to processing this level of liquid, will struggle, and you will be visiting the toilet a little more often than you're used to. This can overload your kidneys and has been known in rare cases to cause kidney damage. It is therefore better to change your lifestyle gradually by increasing the amount of water you drink by an extra pint per day, until eight pints is the norm. Our advice is not to gulp down all six to eight pints of water at once, rather, sip your water gradually throughout the day. In our centre, our lovely Chiropractic assistants keep us hydrated by topping up our glasses of water. If you don't have someone to do this for you, go to work with a two-litre bottle and refill your glass during the day until there's not a drop left. Job done!

Tea and coffee should not be included in your daily water intake allowance. For every cup of coffee or tea you drink, you should drink another glass of water. The reason for this is because both tea and coffee contain varying levels of caffeine. Caffeine is well known for its powers of perking up your brain when tired, but the lesser known fact is that it acts as a diuretic. In other words, it makes you want to urinate more which means that your body is losing precious fluids and is dehydrating.

"But I only drink decaffeinated coffee and teas!" You could be forgiven for thinking that this is the healthier option, but the chemical process of stripping out the caffeine from the coffee beans and tea leaves is, more often than not, worse for your body's toxicity levels than having a weak cup of regular tea or coffee. Alternatively, you could seek out those brands of decaffeinated coffee and teas which boast of being Water Filtered or Swiss Water Filtered. This process involves removing the caffeine over a longer period of time and hence tends to be more expensive, but is much kinder to your body and is a more natural way of de-caffeinating your drinks.

So now you have your Water Filtered decaf coffee or tea in front of you, and you take a sip. Due to the nature of the brew, it's a little too bitter and so you decide to add in a spoonful of sugar and give it a stir. It now tastes much better! Did you know that some studies show that when we ingest sugar, it lights up more spots in our brains than the highly addictive drug, cocaine? That's right —sugar is often said to be even more addictive than cocaine! But sugar isn't illegal. Perhaps it should be, though, as eating too much of this substance over a period of time can lead to your pancreas (the organ which produces insulin) to become overworked. Over time, this damages your pancreas to such an extent that it no longer produces insulin. When a pancreas can no longer produce insulin this results in Type II diabetes along with all the health ramifications that come with being diabetic. This can include heart disease and stroke, nerve damage, diabetic retinopathy (damage to the blood vessels of the eye), kidney disease, and atherosclerosis (the build-up of fatty substances which narrow the blood flow through your blood vessels), which can lead to poor blood circulation throughout the body.

"A-ha," we hear you say, "but I add sweeteners to my drinks, that's not sugar." And yes, you are correct, Sweeteners such as aspartame and sorbitol, to name just a couple, do not work in the same way as natural sugar. When your body breaks them down, one of the byproducts produced is formaldehyde. This chemical has been widely used in the past to preserve the deceased. We are not sure how many people, once aware of this, would choose to ingest formaldehyde. Some studies have also shown that contact with formaldehyde can lead to nerve damage and even cancer, in some cases.

The concern with "fake sugars" and sweeteners are that they are hidden in so many food products. And sometimes, the food labels can be misleading. In the past, if a product was labelled "sugar free," you could bet your bottom dollar that what this actually meant was "contains sweeteners." These days, labels such as "reduced sugar" often also means "contains sweeteners." The list of "sugar free" and "reduced sugar" products is vast, and varies from biscuits to sweets, from chewing gum to sugar replacements. The high consumption of sweeteners or fake sugars is concerning, not just in the form of cordials and squashes, but in fizzy, canned drinks, too. Sadly, a lot of advertising is aimed at those who want to be "healthy," and reduce their calorie intake.

We heard an interesting case study recently about a young male in his late teens who began to develop Multiple Sclerosis-like symptoms. He went from being a normally active young man to one who started to exhibit muscle weakness. This progressed at such a pace that over a period of a few months, he became wheelchair-bound. The scientists were baffled. All scans were coming back as normal. It wasn't until, as a last resort, a nutritionist was added to the medical team. What he found was very interesting. This young man was drinking an enormous amount of fizzy, diet Cola every day. Approximately 4 litres, seven times a week. They decided that the amount of fake sugars being consumed was playing havoc with his nervous system. The "cure" was to stop him drinking diet drinks, and over a period of time, his body did return to normal. There have also been reported cases of people suffering from Fibromyalgia who had symptomatic relief once they stopped ingesting aspartame. Interesting!

Alcohol is another substance to drink in moderation. Not just because it is a toxin and causes liver damage (and in some severe cases, brain damage), but chronic alcohol consumption can lead to osteoporosis (thinning of the bones, making them brittle). In fact, chronic smoking and alcohol consumption not only slows the healing process but is the leading cause of osteopenia in men in the western world. So it is best to predominantly drink filtered water.

Did you know that due to modern day farming methods, today's food tends to be lower in nutrients? In fact, the recommended daily allowance tables that were published way back in 1968 were based on studies from fruits and vegetables farmed less intensively and in better soils. This is particularly true in the case of magnesium. Our soils used to be much higher in magnesium, but modern farming methods have stripped this away. The advice of "an apple a day keeps the doctor away" may have been true back then, but not so much now. If you eat foods that are "in season," then you have a better chance of obtaining some good quality nutrition. Failing that, we advise that you take a good quality food supplement. Not all supplements are created equal, though.

There is evidence to support our belief that food state vitamins and minerals are more effective than laboratory manufactured ones (with the exception of vitamin C). Most supplements that you can buy in supermarkets and popular health food stores tend to be laboratory manufactured. They also tend to be cheaper. So, for example, let's say you decide to take a magnesium supplement from the supermarket. It says magnesium on the bottle but not the magic words "food state" or "whole food." This means that each capsule taken does contain a substance with the same chemical formula as magnesium but not in a form that the body recognises. It passes through the body without being absorbed, and out the other end. With Food State tablets, the vitamin is grown in plants, such as broccoli, so that the body recognises it as food. It follows the same pathways as food does and is absorbed by the body normally. Also check to make sure that the coatings of your tablets contain natural, not manufactured ingredients, as some contain substances not good for us -such as fake sugars- and some contain substances which are known to be carcinogenic.

VITAMIN/ MINERAL:	FUNCTION:	DEFICIENCY SYMPTOMS:
Calcium	Helps build strong bones, blood clotting and muscle contractions (including the heart). When taking calcium it's important to take magnesium as well, as they affect how each other works. Studies suggest a 2:1 calcium to magnesium ratio to avoid osteoporosis (brittle bones)	Muscle cramps and weakness, weakened bone strength, bleeding and bruising easily.
Vitamin D	Vitamin D is also important in calcium absorption hence they are normally taken together.	Painful bones, and muscle weakness. Decreased bone density, which, if left, can lead to osteoporosis and fractures.
Magnesium	Is important for good nerve and muscle function	Muscle cramps, fascial "tics", poor sleep and chronic pain
Selenium	Is important for thyroid gland function, DNA production and protecting the body from free radicals and infections. There are very low quantities in our food	Hypothyroidism, extreme fatigue, hair loss, goitre, mental fatigue or brain fog, lowered immunity -- and can be linked to recurring miscarriage.

	when grown in soil that still contains it. Very few people get enough this way. Selenium helps to convert thyroxine (T4) to its more active form, triiodothyronine (T3).	
Vitamin B complex	Important for energy metabolism, nerve function, eyes, skin, and digestion	Anaemia, balance problems, numbness and tingling in hands (also a symptom of excess vitamin B6), legs or feet, difficulty in thinking and reasoning or memory loss.
Zinc	Helps the immune system to work properly. It plays a part in cell division, cell growth and in healing wounds. It helps to breakdown carbohydrates. Zinc is also needed for smell and taste.	Hair loss, diarrhoea, eye and skin sores, loss of appetite, weight loss, slow wound healing, decreased ability to taste food, and brain fog.
Iron	A lack of iron causes a decrease of oxygenated blood in the body due to a reduction in the protein, haemoglobin.	Fatigue, weakness, racing heart, breathlessness, headaches, cold hands/feet, inflammation, sore tongue, brittle nails, poor appetite-especially in the young, or an attraction to starchy foods

The table above shows common vitamins and minerals, how these help to keep the body healthy-and what can happen if your diet is low in them.

It is interesting to note that when it comes to checking thyroid function, blood tests can often come back as inconclusive, or "normal." One reason for this could be because the levels of TSH (Thyroid Stimulating Hormone) and the thyroid hormone T4 (thyroxine) seem to be tested more than the T3 (tyrosine) levels. T3 can often be low and result in thyroid dysfunction. Interestingly, the body converts T4 to T3 using Selenium. This is why we frequently recommend a Selenium supplement.Another reason can be because the levels of what is classed as "normal" are very broad.

The important thing to realise when you decide to supplement your diet is that it can actually take up to three months to rebuild your body's stores and for the supplement to make a difference, so consistency is key.

Sometimes, though, no matter how diligent you are at eating a balanced diet, there are certain foods that some people cannot digest effectively. There are studies which show that there could be a link between a pregnant mother's diet in her last trimester, as well as the first few weeks of breast feeding, to food intolerances in her children, particularly if the mother eats those foods that have proven to be common allergens. For these individuals, there are certain foods to which they are either intolerant, or in some cases, severely allergic. In this chapter we will be covering the more common food intolerances; the ones we encounter time and time again here in our centre.

Number one has to be dairy, and by this we mean not only the obvious suspects such as milk, cheese and butter, but also those hidden ones in breads, cakes, biscuits, and even some crisps! For those who find dairy hard to digest, symptoms can present, such as lethargy, tiredness, over-production of phlegm, coughing or sneezing fits, sinusitis and eczema. For most, it is the milk sugar called lactose that is the culprit. When searching for a good source of natural calcium, most people think of milk. Cow's milk contains calcium, but not in a form the body can break down and utilise easily. It is therefore better to switch to dairy-free alternatives such as coconut, almond, rice, oat, or hemp milk. Personally, we are not huge fans of soya milk, as its production is potentially harmful to the environment, and we already eat a lot of products that contain hidden levels. Soya is also high in plant hormones called phyto-oestrogens. Science is unsure yet about whether plant oestrogens are harmful to our health-particularly reproductive health.

Calcium is also present in good levels in dark, green vegetables. Adult cows don't drink their own milk, yet they continue to have strong bones and adequate calcium in their bodies. This means you don't need to drink milk to ensure you are ingesting enough calcium. If you are taking a supplement, it is important to remember that calcium can displace the levels of magnesium in your body, resulting in a magnesium deficiency and possible symptoms such as cramp (whilst vitamin D helps the body to absorb calcium) this is why it is advisable to seek professional advice before taking any supplement.

The second most common intolerance we see is wheat. Usually, it is an intolerance to gluten, a protein found in wheat. Gluten is found in breads, cereals, cakes, biscuits and pastas. If you are intolerant to gluten, you can suffer from symptoms which include lethargy and tiredness, eczema, bloating, bouts of diarrhoea and constipation, and abdominal cramps, to name but a few. Since gluten inflames the bowels, symptoms often follow that of Irritable Bowel Syndrome (IBS). For those diagnosed with a more serious reaction to gluten, the diagnosis of Coeliac disease may be made.

Recent studies are beginning to draw strong correlations between chronic inflammation of the bowels and lower back pain. What is believed to be happening is that the inflammation of the intestines, switches off the muscles that lie close to the spine. With these core muscles fatiguing, the spine loses some structural support and is then more prone to injury and pain.

So it might be easier to stick to nature's alternatives, such as oat-based cereals like the classic porridge. You are also fine to eat rice and potatoes.

Surprisingly, many people have an intolerance to onions and tomatoes. More so in their raw form than their cooked states. Symptoms include lethargy and tiredness, acid reflux and heartburn, burping, bloating, and abdominal cramping. In fact, if you consider the ingredients in a traditional Margarita pizza, then you have a handy reminder of what to avoid. You have wheat in its crust, dairy in the melted cheese on top, and onions and tomatoes in the sauce covering the pizza base.

One particular gentleman we saw came to us with chronic lower back pain coupled with terrible bouts of indigestion, and he couldn't eat anything without getting heartburn. It was really starting to get him down as this was taking the joy out of dinner dates with his wife.The specialists he had seen were baffled and none of their suggestions seemed to work and he had been told that he would need to take antacids for life.

So we started, as we always do, with realigning his spine. This was to reduce irritation to the nerves linked to his diaphragm, stomach and digestive organs. We also then worked hard on loosening up his diaphragm with a diaphragm release technique. This worked really well. We also suggested that he completely cut out onions from his diet. This combined approach saw his indigestion improve, as well as the back pain he had initially come to see us for. He now chooses to attend the centre regularly, in order to keep his heartburn at bay.

Another particularly interesting case springs to mind. This lady presented to us with lower back pain and a secondary complaint of irritable bowel syndrome. She had undergone operations in the past, which had resulted in sections of her bowel being removed due to a previous history of bowel cancer. She could not go out at night due to the fact that she needed to be on the toilet every night for three hours. Spending that amount of time on the toilet each night was not helping her lower back at all. After an examination, we decided to take some x-rays of her lower back, to rule out any sinister causes for her pain. The X-ray revealed a severe scoliosis with a loss of bone density (osteoporosis), and degenerative changes of a severe nature. We knew we had to help this lady. She could not continue to live that way. We knew the nerves were being irritated in the lower back, and we also knew that this was really not helping the way her bowels functioned. We set about working on her body as a whole, working particularly around her lower back and pelvis to reduce the pressure on the nerves enabling the bowels to function better. After a few months of care, this patient's lower back pain reduced dramatically and her time on the toilet was down to an hour a night. This gave her a much better quality of life and she was able to contemplate evenings out, without having to worry about three-hour trips to the bathroom.

We do see our fair share of people who are allergic to peanuts and other nuts. Nuts do tend to elicit a more severe reaction (called anaphylaxis) in those susceptible. Symptoms include wheezing and difficulty breathing, light headedness, increased heart rate and sweating, and in some cases, unconsciousness and even death. Other foods that can cause this reaction in some are eggs, fish, shellfish, and some fruits.

Over the years, we have had the pleasure of attending many a Chiropractic conference. One such conference happened to be held in one of those rather lovely airport hotels adjacent to Heathrow. This hotel used to offer a tasty buffet lunch, but for some reason, this was unavailable the weekend we were there, and so we decided to take a short walk down the road to the next hotel. A feast awaited us: a wide variety of salads, soups, cheeses, fruits and savouries. We couldn't wait to tuck in. Little did we know that in a few moments' time, Wendy's throat would start to constrict, her breathing would become more difficult and her eyelids would puff up, restricting her vision. The culprit? Under-ripe, freshly-cut pineapple rings, which Wendy had sampled. Unfortunately for her, as it turns out, pineapple contains the enzyme, Bromelain, to which she is mildly allergic. So now, Wendy is slightly more selective in her choice of fruit!

What is also important is not just what you choose to fuel your body with but when you choose to eat it, and how much of it you eat. Eating habits are instilled in us from when we are young, so empower yourself now by making good, healthy choices. Fad diets are unsustainable. Keeping a food diary for a week is a great way to check your nutritional journey and helps us make better, future choices. Humans are drawn to sweet foods as they provide "easy, quick energy" which was advantageous when we were being chased by woolly mammoths and sabre-toothed tigers. This is the same reason we are drawn to fats as they are rich in calories. But by keeping your metabolism high and your blood sugars level, you won't go hungry.

Start your day with complex carbohydrates and lean proteins which take longer to break down and give a slower release of energy, making you feel fuller for longer. Foods such as porridge and other oat-based cereals combined with a non-dairy milk (for protein) and three portions of fruit is great. Try and eat breakfast within an hour of waking up. In an ideal world, we should be eating five equally-sized meals a day to maintain a steady metabolism. If you can't do this, then stick to three main meals a day, but intersperse these with transition meals, not snacks. A transitional meal should be a handful-sized portion of protein coupled with some fibre. So, for example, this could be some nuts or a non-dairy yoghurt with some dried fruit or berries.

Talking about food portions, when having your main meals, divide your plate into five sections, one fifth being the equivalent of a handful. One fifth should contain protein, this can be plant or animal, so for example this could be red meat, poultry, fish, eggs, dairy, lentils, beans and pulses. Three-fifths should contain fibre, for example fruits, vegetables or salads. Fill the remaining fifth of your plate with complex carbohydrates such as whole grains, oats and rice. Try and make sure that you eat your last meal at least two hours before you go to bed to allow yourself enough time to digest it. Your body doesn't want to be, nor should it be, multitasking whilst you are asleep. Like most things in life, if you stick to this for three weeks it should become a habit. Healthy habits lead to healthy lifestyles.

Chapter summary:

You are what you eat and drink. Your body is composed mostly of water. Ensure you drink a minimum of two litres of water a day and limit your intake of caffeinated, alcoholic, and sugary drinks. Common food intolerances are gluten, dairy, tomatoes and onions. Changing farming methods have had a knock-on effect on what our foods contain, so it may be important to supplement our diet with food state minerals. Divide your plate into fifths when eating: one fifth protein, one fifth carbohydrate, three-fifths fibre-containing foods.

CHAPTER 8:
EXERCISE CAN BE BAD FOR YOU

Okay, we admit it, the title of this chapter is perhaps misleading. We all know that our bodies were designed to move and moving is good for us and our health. In fact, it is recommended that we do at least 30 minutes of moderate exercise three times a week; exercise that gets us slightly out of breath so that holding a conversation is difficult.

Exercise gets your blood pumping, burns calories, and releases those happy hormones called endorphins. You can do it on your own or in groups, and it is a great way of meeting people who will keep you motivated. Exercising also stimulates postural receptors in your joints. It is these signals which are said to stimulate the brain. So exercising doesn't just stimulate the body but the brain as well. People who exercise regularly tend to have lower cholesterol and better cardiovascular systems. Exercise also helps to stimulate digestion and improve bowel movements by decreasing the time food takes to travel through the colon. The shorter the time the food spends in the large intestine, the less time it takes your body to absorb water from your stools. Firmer stools are more difficult to pass and this helps to stimulate peristalsis (contractions) of the bowels, resulting in excretion of the stool.

But are you choosing the right exercise for you? Did you know that for some, certain exercises are considered to be counter-productive, whilst some exercises would benefit most people?

In this chapter, we are going to cover the most regularly prescribed stretches and exercises that we give to those who seek our care here in the centre. We will also provide you with a heads-up with regards to the exercises we tend to ask people to avoid.

Let's start with what you should be doing first. The large majority of people who seek our help tend to do so because they are in some sort of pain or discomfort. Whilst loading the washing machine, or even sneezing, they may have put their back out, or they may have been reversing their car down the road, locked their neck, and subsequently been unable to return their head to a forward position. Whatever the final straw was, the vertebral bones in their spine have become misaligned, resulting in swelling of the nearby tissues, which has then placed pressure on the exiting spinal nerves, resulting in pain.

Now we get asked this question an awful lot: "Should I use a heat pad or an ice pack to soothe the area?" We tend to reply to this question with another question, "if you were to sprain your ankle, what would you use —hot or cold?" and the usual answer goes something like this: "cold, of course!" Why is that? The answer is that when you sprain your ankle, swelling occurs due to the inflammation of the tissues. We place ice on the area because not only is it a fantastic, natural painkiller by numbing the area directly at the source of the problem, but it also works very well as a natural anti-inflammatory, reducing swelling and aiding the healing process. So the reasons you place ice on your sprained ankle are the same reasons you should use it on your back or neck to reduce the inflammation.

When you place something cold on the body, it causes the local blood vessels to constrict, which in turn reduces blood flow to the area. Reduced blood flow means less blood and less swelling. Placing heat on the site adds heat to an area that is already inflamed. So, although heat can feel nice, it is not as effective as ice.

One day, a lovely lady came to see us. She had been suffering from lower back pain and had seen all those television adverts advertising heat packs. Prior to examining her, we asked her to get changed, keep her underwear on and then to put on an examination gown over the top. We couldn't believe it when we opened up the back of her gown to see her spine. The lower half of her back was covered in what looked to be the strangest, red-raw rash we had ever seen. Strange, because it appeared to have a particular pattern to it. A pattern of criss-crossed lines producing multiple diamond shapes. The oddest thing was that this "rash" was not itchy or sore and this lady had no knowledge of its existence. It was only on further questioning that we both realised what it was. She had been filling up her favourite hot water bottle with boiling hot water from the kettle. Then, with nothing covering it, she'd been placing it directly onto her lower back, thus increasing blood flow to the skin, matching the pattern on her hot water bottle. The skin did recover over time but it is a lesson in being mindful when using heat and/or ice.

If you choose to use ice you need to select something really cold that has been living in your freezer and not your fridge. Don't use a hard, plastic picnic brick that has been loitering at the bottom of your freezer. It's too rigid. It is better to use something malleable, i.e. something that will mould to the contours of your body. Specialist gel-filled ice packs, crushed ice cubes in a plastic bag, and bags of frozen peas or sweetcorn work well. Make sure you can differentiate between your food and your medical aids —label your peas and sweetcorn as "ice packs," as it's easy to defrost, freeze, and defrost them again —let's not add food poisoning to your list of symptoms! Whatever you decide to use, wrap it up in something thin, like a tea-towel or pillow case to avoid ice burns. Do not use a hand towel as this will be too thick, and do not place the ice pack directly onto your skin. Additionally, it is really important that you correctly place the ice pack.

If icing the neck, remember to place the pack in the middle, down the back of the neck. Do not allow the cold to cover the side of your neck. We learned early on to give this advice. One of our patients told us she had stopped icing it as it had been making her feel faint. After a little bit of detective work, we realised that because she felt like her pain was originating from the side of her neck and shoulder region, this was where she had been placing her ice pack. Unfortunately, this is also the location of a major artery for the brain; the carotid artery. When you place something that cold on an artery, it constricts, thus reducing blood flow —and in this case, reducing blood flow to the brain, which was causing this woman to feel faint. So, for neck complaints, please remember to place the ice pack onto the back of the neck and not onto the side or front.

For lower back complaints, place the covered ice pack across the lower half of the back at about belt level. To avoid ice burns, we advise removing the ice pack after 20 minutes. Repeat this process three times a day, and continue until either the pain has eased, or your clinician tells you otherwise.

Once you have used your ice pack correctly and reduced the inflammation, you will feel less pain and be able to move more easily, but how mobile and flexible are you? Well, let's talk you through some easy-to-do tests you can try at home.

Can you touch your toes? No cheating, now! Stand with your feet hip distance apart. Bend forward and slide your hands down over your knees and see how far down your shins you can reach. Can you touch your toes now? If you can't get within ten centimetres of the floor, then you may need to increase your flexibility by stretching out your back and hamstring muscles, and by getting the bones of your lower spine and pelvis better aligned.

Lying on your back, lift one leg at a time, nice and straight, and as high as you can. Do your legs reach 90 degrees either side? If not, it's well worth your while asking a musculoskeletal expert such as a Chiropractor, Osteopath or an Osteomyologist to check you over.

To check how flexible your shoulders are, reach up and over your head with one hand and try and scratch between your shoulder blades. With the other hand, reach behind your back, and see if you can touch the fingers of the hand scratching your shoulder blades. Now swap sides and repeat. If your fingers are nowhere near each other, then the flexibility of your shoulders could do with being looked at.

Now sit on the floor with your back resting against the wall. Bend your knees so that your feet and knees are side-by-side and together. Keeping your feet together, let your knees fall outwards and towards the floor. Do your knees touch the ground? How far off the ground are they? If you cannot get your knees over halfway to the floor, then the flexibility of your hip region may need examining.

How easy is it for you to look over your left and right shoulders? Fix your gaze on a specific point directly behind you. You should be able to see this point equally over both right and left shoulders. Most people soon realise that they can actually look further behind them on one side more than the other.

Wendy's mum certainly found this out the hard way when Wendy was only six years old, living in a house situated on a hill. Access to the main road was via a long, brick driveway, which ran straight down to the road from the carport. With no turning circle, this meant that you drove up the driveway and then had to reverse back down, whilst looking over one shoulder. It took about ten years of repeatedly doing this to create some degenerative changes in her neck. Then one day after arriving at the bottom of the brick driveway, Wendy's mum found she couldn't turn her head back round to the front. Her neck was stuck! Luckily for her, one of her friends advised her to "go and see this guy", who turned out to be a Chiropractor. Wendy went along with her, and although she didn't get to witness the adjustment that her mum received to her neck -she was too busy playing with the wooden cars and building blocks in the welcome area -she does remember her Mum being able to swivel her neck much better afterwards. Wendy's mum has been a huge advocate of Chiropractic care ever since, and it definitely helped inspire her daughter to join this great profession.

Now you have a good idea of how flexible you are (or not), what follows below is a selection of stretches for the neck and lower back that we have found to be beneficial for the vast majority of people who come and seek our help.

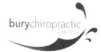

Our Top Stretches
for a more flexible you.

Knee to Chest - Lower Back Stretch
Muscles worked: Erector spinae

how to do it
& what it should look like

1 Lie on a bed, on your back.   Image A
    a) Bring your legs up towards your chest.
    b) Wrap both hands around your knees.
2 Slowly pull your knees toward your chest until you feel a stretch in   Image B
  your lower back.
    a) Keep your knees and feet together.
    b) Keep your head and upper trunk flat on the bed.
3 Hold for 12 seconds, release, and **repeat three times**.
4 Repeat twice daily.

Cat Stretch & Prayer Pose - Lower Back Stretch
Muscles worked: Latissimus dorsi, erector spinae, rhomboids

how to do it
& what it should look like

Starting Position - Come down on your hands and knees with your hands   Image A
shoulder-width apart, knees hip-width apart, and keep your back flat (spine neutral).

Action - Engage your abdominals as if pulling your navel towards your spine, and
round your back towards the ceiling. Allow your head and neck to fall naturally
between the arms.

1 Assume the same pose as for the cat stretch.   Image B
2 Keep your hands on the floor in front of you and ease backwards so that your
  bottom rests on your heels.
3 Lower your body towards the floor, allowing your hands to slide forwards (whilst
  keeping your bottom on your heels).
4 Feel the stretch in your lower back and hold for 12 seconds.
5 Release, and resume cat pose. Repeat A, followed by B, 3 times in a row.
6 Repeat twice daily.

Neck Stretches
Muscles worked: SCM, scalene, trapezius, levator scapulae, splenius capitis, splenius cervicis, rhomboid

how to do it
& what it should look like

1 Hold the top of your head with your right hand, just above your left ear   Image A
2 Gently pull your head sideways so that your right ear moves towards your right shoulder
3 Hold for **12 seconds**, release and **repeat 3 times**
4 Now repeat for the left side
5 Repeat twice daily

1 Hold the top of your head with your right hand so that your elbow is in line   Image B
  with your nose
2 Rotate your head 40 degrees and gently pull downwards
3 Hold for **12 seconds**, release and **repeat 3 times**
4 Now repeat with your left hand
5 Repeat twice daily

1 Stretch your arms out in front of you & clasp one hand on top of the other   Image C
2 Gently reach out so that you feel your shoulder blades stretching away from each other
3 Gently lower your head downwards so that your chin moves towards your chest
4 Hold for **12 seconds**.
5 Repeat 2-4 times

ALWAYS REMEMBER!
1 Hold each stretch for the magical stretching time of 12 seconds 2 Do not bounce 3 Stretch to slight tension, not pain 4 If ANY stretch results in pain/ worsens your pain STOP IMMEDIATELY! 5 Then consult your Clinician on how to proceed

Complete the stretches at least 2-3 times daily.

t: 0161 763 1700 | Bury Chiropractic Ltd | Exchange House | 39 Knowsley Street | Bury, Lancs BL9 0ST

The image on the previous page gives examples of some the most common stretches we give to help alleviate back and neck symptoms.

Imagine that you are easing back into exercise after an injury, or that you are new to a regular exercise routine. In this scenario, we always recommend that you start with walking. Walking is low impact and is safe for pretty much everyone. Wear comfortable, flat trainers, walking boots or shoes. Walking is great for the discs in your spine. This is because the discs rely on the movement of the bones above and below them to pump nutrients in and take waste products away. Walking creates this movement, thus aiding the healing process. It is mainly for this reason that walking, and not, as in the past, bed rest, is now recommended for people suffering from mechanical lower back pain. If you can, time your walk for the morning. This is because your early morning walk could positively affect your blood pressure by lowering the hormone, cortisol. Cortisol is sometimes referred to as the "stress hormone" and it has peaks and troughs throughout the day, so exercising during the peaks can be beneficial. Most people experience peaks in their cortisol levels between 8-9am, 12-1pm, and 5:30-6:30pm. A good 15-20 minutes of brisk walking on a daily basis at these peak times is a great start.

Another form of exercise that we recommend is swimming. Swimming is non-weight-bearing and so is gentle on your joints. There are some things to consider, though, before you choose to add swimming to your new, healthy lifestyle. Stick to doing backstroke. In our day-to-day lives, we are constantly working with things in front of us, whether that be bending over a laptop, driving our cars, or preparing the evening meal. The great thing about backstroke is that it makes our bodies perform in the totally opposite way, working those muscles not often utilised. This not only improves your posture, but works those muscles closest to your spine, the core muscles.

Be careful to avoid breaststroke. The posture you adopt when swimming breaststroke overarches the neck and lower back, as well as putting a strain on your hip and knee joints. We tend to advise using this technique as a recovery stroke to be used once every ten lengths or so. Make sure that when you do, that you are mindful of your posture, that your head goes under the water, and that you really stretch forwards and glide between each stroke.

Front crawl, or freestyle swimming, is fine as long as your head is in the water, that you kick mainly from the hips and not the knees, and that you turn your head to alternate sides when taking a breath. If you breathe every three strokes, you will get into a great rhythm and have the bonus of using both sides of your neck, avoiding too much repetition on one side, which can create irritation in the neck joints.

If you are looking for a fitness class, then we recommend trying Pilates or Yoga. Yoga is great for improving flexibility, and Pilates is great for training the core muscles. Just be careful to avoid instructions which involve over-arching backwards, as this can quite often irritate the facet joints and surrounding tissues in the lower back and neck.

Many people who come to see us want to return to running. Unfortunately, running is classed as a high impact sport as far as the joints of your body are concerned. The axial compression caused whilst running with joints that are already stuck will only serve to inflame and exacerbate the area. Once your joints have been aligned and the swelling has gone, you may still want to return to running. If so, you can reduce the impact it has on your joints. Firstly, consider your running shoes. How many miles have you run in them? Over time, they will have become worn, and you will have lost the good support they used to give you. Running shoes should be changed every 300 to 500 miles. Once your feet are supported, you need to consider what surfaces you are running on. Running on hard ground such as roads and pavements will send more shock waves through your joints than if you run on softer ground such as grass or on a treadmill. Try and run on softer ground, and if you are running on the roads then switch to grassy verges whenever you can.

Many of us are members of a gym. We do have people who come to us after overdoing it in the gym, using the wrong equipment, or by using the right equipment with a poor technique. The two main culprits for causing problems tend to be the rowing machine and the vertical stepper. If you do not get someone who knows how to set the rowing machine up for you specifically, or if you are not trained in the correct rowing technique, this piece of equipment is best avoided. Used incorrectly, it places huge strain on your lower back, hips and knees. The stepper, if used incorrectly, can also cause strain on your knees, pelvis and lower back. There are lots of other great pieces of gym equipment, so missing out these two shouldn't impact on your gym fitness. For a cardiovascular workout, we tend to advise using the cross trainers, treadmills on the flat, and exercise bikes.

There is something we have started to notice more and more, which only used to apply to regular gym-goers and semi-professional sportsmen, and that is the use of technology strapped to the chests or wrists. These devices monitor the pulse rate, calories burned, steps taken, and/or the distance travelled. Today, more and more people are using them as watches as well as monitoring devices, and we are not entirely convinced this is healthy for you. Your body, due to the electrical impulses produced by your nervous system, generates its own electromagnetic field. When you strap an electronic monitoring device, which is generating its own electromagnetic field, onto your wrist, or strap it to your chest, we believe it has the potential to play havoc with your body's natural magnetic field and we just don't know if there are any long-term health benefits or risks of using equipment like this. We would therefore recommend that you do not have it permanently on you. If you do, we would advise to limit its usage as much as possible and only use it when exercising.

Either that, or you could wear it in combination with an energy-rebalancing product, such as an Energy Dot. Energy dots are low power magnets. They are programmed with a naturally occurring bio-energetic information signature, which is stored in a similar way that your bank information is stored on the magnetic strip of your bank card. The powerful resonance held by the dot acts like a tuning fork on electromagnetic fields and retunes man-made electromagnetic fields to a more natural harmony, via a process called Entrainment. The human body recognises these retuned emissions as being in synchronisation with its natural healthy state. Since the body is now in harmony, it no longer has to fight these emissions, and electro-stress is then relieved.

Chapter summary:

The right type of exercise is good for you, e.g. walking. Avoid using the rowing machine and stepping machine in the gym and change your trainers regularly. The correct use of an ice pack is effective at reducing symptoms when placed appropriately. Limit the use of monitoring devices that could potentially affect your body's electro-magnetic field.

CHAPTER 9:
SURGERY SHOULD BE THE LAST RESORT

In our opinion, surgery should always be used as a last resort. It's invasive, and an area that has been operated on will rarely function as well as it used to.

Surgery will always leave varying amounts of scar tissue behind; scar tissue can cause problems and change the function of that particular part of the body. That said, some operations can be lifesavers. We are not advocating the refusal of life-saving operations such as heart surgery, for example, but we have seen many people over the years who have had operations to correct immobility and pain and have, sadly, suffered side effects.

Their journey will most likely have started by taking painkillers for a particular symptom. Over time, they may have found that those painkillers had done little or nothing for their problem. Further trips to the GP meant that diagnostic tests such as MRI scans or X-rays were undertaken. Whilst awaiting the results of those to determine the cause of their symptoms, their painkillers may well have caused further unwanted side effects and may not have even had the desired result of reducing their initial symptoms. In this scenario, it is likely that further medications were then prescribed to help combat those side effects.

Once the cause of the problem was established, exercises may then have been prescribed, which can at times make the symptoms feel worse rather than better. At this point the conclusion is often reached that the only option left is to undergo surgery.

It is likely that the patient was informed that the symptom or symptoms they are suffering from are the result of arthritis, and that eventually, they will need a joint replacement. It may feel as though there is nothing else which can be done other than wait for the arthritis to become severe enough to be operated upon, and that a replacement is inevitable. But this need not be the case. Something *can* be done.

The worst thing to do is to ignore a symptom or neglect it, waiting until the pain becomes unbearable. Pain can cause you to alter your natural movement patterns and it's this that can place pressure on other parts of the body, resulting in premature degeneration, or even accelerate degeneration in secondary sites.

For example, walking around with a limp for many years because of a degenerative hip can cause the knee on the opposite leg to lock up and become arthritic. Arthritic knees then result in further altered walking patterns, causing more pressure to build up in the hip joints. Please seek help before the only option available to you in this scenario is both a knee and a hip replacement.

Indeed, this is what happened to a lady we knew. She loved to ride horses and was always on the go. Over the years, she developed problems with her left knee. This knee gradually began to tighten up and she started to lose flexion, or the ability to bend it. This resulted in a walking pattern that involved rolling from side-to-side rather than one that was balanced and correct. The knock-on effect was the development of right hip, lower back and buttock symptoms. It became so much of a problem that it stopped her doing the one thing she loved to do: riding her horse. A lower back and hip X-ray revealed severe degeneration of the right hip, and a joint replacement was recommended. She had the surgery and was back horse riding within two or three months. However, the left knee pain and restriction was worsening, and the lower back was still troublesome. She then found that she developed shoulder pain, all on her right side.

This was because the left knee pain and restriction she had originally started with hadn't been addressed. When symptoms are ignored, they can continue, and even worsen. The best time to do something is when a problem begins.

Indeed, we have also seen a similar case (and many more like this) where a lady attended our centre, complaining of left shoulder pain and left-sided lower back pain. She had been born with a dislocated hip that had gone undiagnosed for years, but by her 30s, she decided enough was enough and that she wanted to have a hip replacement. Surgery was performed, and her hip pain eased. However, the operation had left her with a 2-3-inch difference in one leg and caused her to waddle, which over a period of time, resulted in lower back and shoulder pain. We worked on levelling out her leg lengths by working on her pelvis and lower back and focused on loosening up her neck to free off the nerves going to the shoulder. This lady responded really nicely to care and continues to receive adjustments on a regular basis to help maintain the progress she made.

You may think that surgery is the answer to all your problems and that once you have recovered from surgery, the area will remain perfect forever. As mentioned in the beginning of our book, here in the UK, the National Health Service is there for people when they need it and there isn't a charge to use it. It's paid for by National Insurance contributions, so in many cases, the NHS feels like it's "free" to us. When something is perceived as being free, less of a value is placed upon it.

We recently overheard a woman talking in the gym about a knee operation she'd had. She had been told to avoid running, cycling and any impact type exercise for at least six weeks after her operation, to allow her body enough time to recover and heal. As she had felt fine a week or two afterwards, she decided she would go to the gym and do some spinning (an energetic cycling class lasting approximately 40 minutes). As she'd had no negative reaction after it, she then decided to try running. She then went spinning again. Again, she felt fine and within two weeks post-operation and exercising, she was back to doing everything in the gym that she wanted to do and had been doing previously. Now, speaking from experience, we know she hadn't allowed her body sufficient time to recover. The knee was still weak, the body was still repairing and we feared for her knee in the long term. We also worried about future problems due to an inadequate recovery time post-operation. Would she have acted differently if she'd had to pay the surgeon thousands of pounds directly? Possibly. It's hard to know. Would she have acted differently if she had to pay for follow-up visits and a further operation? It's hard to attribute value to something you have not paid for.

Although there is a certain amount of recuperation time involved with any operation, once you have recovered, you have recovered. There tends to be less emphasis placed on doing things to help yourself, and also less motivation to do these things once the perceived cause of the problem has been rectified. Other forms of care, whether that be Acupuncture, Osteopathy or Chiropractic, for example, involve a time and energy commitment as well as a financial one. Time and energy to make your appointments, and money to pay for them. We all lead busy lives and time is precious. It's hard to snatch 30 minutes here and 30 minutes there.

Sadly, in our time in private practice as Chiropractors, we have seen many cases of failed surgical procedures. Carpal tunnel syndrome is one such example. This is where a nerve that comes from the neck and into the wrist becomes irritated, or "trapped" at the wrist, resulting in muscle weakness, tingling, numbness and pain. Surgery involves freeing up the nerve at the site of entrapment within the wrist, thereby relieving the symptoms. This operation can fail, because quite often, the influence of the neck on the wrist is overlooked. If nerves are irritated in the neck, they can cause similar symptoms in the wrist. This is because the nerves in the neck supply the wrist and when they are irritated, they can cause symptoms similar to those of carpal tunnel syndrome.

One particular patient we saw decided to consult a surgeon for an opinion on problems he was having with his wrist. His pain was not severe but as it was in his right wrist, his writing wrist, it was frustrating for him.

The surgeon decided to operate, and the patient was left with a nice scar and symptoms which settled down for a year or so but returned with a vengeance and worse than ever a year after that. An examination of his nervous system and orthopaedic tests revealed that his neck was not functioning well. Indeed, this person's job involved a lot of driving and computer work, which was placing a lot of pressure on the nerves in his neck. After working on the neck and the rest of the body by adjusting the bones and enabling the body to do what it does best- heal itself, the symptoms settled, and a further operation was avoided.

That is not to say that all surgical procedures fail. Indeed, there are many cases where an operation has been the only way of resolving a problem. However, the most common musculoskeletal operations we have seen are hip replacements, knee replacements, or arthroscopies and carpal tunnel surgeries.

With the hip replacements, we have seen many go on to suffer from a lot of lower back pain and neck pain. This is often because a replacement has left them with a leg length discrepancy that they are then having to walk around on. Hip replacements are not custom-made or bespoke. There are different standard sizes to fit different people, but generally, what you are given as a replacement will never be as good as what you were initially born with. A person who needs a replacement, or who has had one, walks about and moves differently. They try to avoid putting undue pressure on the painful hip, but in doing so, cause an imbalance to develop in the spine. Over a period of time this imbalance can cause an "s" shape, or *scoliosis*, to form in the spine. A scoliosis is when a straight spine viewed from the front, or from behind, becomes "S" shaped. This "S" shape can then draw a leg "up," resulting in an apparent leg length difference. The new hip is either then fitted with that "S" shape in place, further perpetuating that leg length difference, or there becomes a leg length difference with the new hip in place. Walking about like this causes further problems elsewhere in the body: in the opposite hip, lower back, or even the neck. Historically, hip replacements only used to last approximately ten years, but as advances have been made, hip replacements now tend to be less intrusive and last longer.

Conversely, we have seen women born with hip dislocations that weren't diagnosed until years later, who have been told they will need a replacement in the future because of the joint being so restricted. In these cases, we have worked on loosening up the hips and rest of the body. In all cases we have been able to increase the range of motion or movement in the hips which have enabled these patients to walk better, have more energy and less pain, and in some cases, the recommended hip operation has been no longer needed. This always leaves us thinking that it's better to seek help first prior to undertaking an operation on an area. In our opinion, surgery should always be a last resort and not the first port of call.

We commonly come across disc "bulges." If a disc has bulged in the spine, to such an extent that it's impinging on one of the nerves exiting the spine, a spinal fusion operation may be recommended. This is where part of the disc is removed and the vertebrae above and below this level can be fused with metal rods. The lower back or Lumbar spine is designed to mainly move forwards and backwards. The individual spinal segments do not move all that much by themselves, but it's the combined movement of all the vertebrae in the lower back which gives the lower back its global range of motion or movement, and allows you to touch your toes, for example. When you fuse two vertebrae together, you decrease the global range of movement which that particular area of the spine controls, and the rest of the spine then has to pick up the slack. This creates stress further up the spine and onto other parts of the body.

There is a place for drugs. Drugs are great for end of life care and in accidents and emergencies. They are good for acute, short-term problems, but they are not a long-term solution. Pain serves as a signal and stops you from doing activities that aggravate a symptom or condition. For example, if bending causes lower back pain, and the drugs numb this pain, allowing you to bend more, further aggravating your condition, is this serving you?

Imagine a fire alarm is going off in a building. There is a fire. Would you want someone to come and remove the batteries from the smoke alarm so you couldn't hear the ringing, or would you want someone to come and put the fire out? Painkillers numb the pain but they don't correct the problem. In this scenario, they stop the ringing of the fire alarm, even though the fire is still there and growing. What you would really want is for someone to come and put that fire out so the subsequent ringing stops never to return again. This is what Chiropractic care enables the body to do: it puts the fire out for it never to return again. Painkillers mask symptoms and allow fires to develop.

We believe Chiropractic care should be the first port of call for any problem, followed by drugs, and surgery should only be considered once all the other options have been exhausted. There are always options even once surgery has been performed but surgery inevitably leaves scar tissue behind. You can still seek Chiropractic care following surgery, and once the surgeon has given the all-clear to proceed, walking is a great exercise. It's low impact, and good for the discs within the spine. Core exercises are vital. These keep all the core muscles around the spine and joints strong so that when you come to do any physical activity, injury is less likely. Yoga and Pilates are also great for strengthening up the core muscles. Stretching is very important as there will be some tightness following a period of immobility, and Chiropractic is great for removing any nerve interference and for enabling the body to heal itself.

Chapter summary:

Surgery is invasive and should always be the last resort. Ignoring symptoms inevitably means causing additional problems for yourself further down the line. Chiropractic care enables the body to heal itself by helping to balance the body and restore function and can prevent the need for surgery. It can also be used post-operatively but should always be the first port of call, in our opinion.

Printed in Poland
by Amazon Fulfillment
Poland Sp. z o.o., Wrocław

51135216R00072